D1524736

# DR. SEBI

# ALKALINE & ANTI-INFLAMMATORY

# DIET

## The 30-Step Transition Action Plan for Beginners

--------------------------------------------------------------

## With Recipes, Meal Plans and More

## By

# Kerri M. Williams

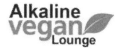

www.alkalineveganlounge.com

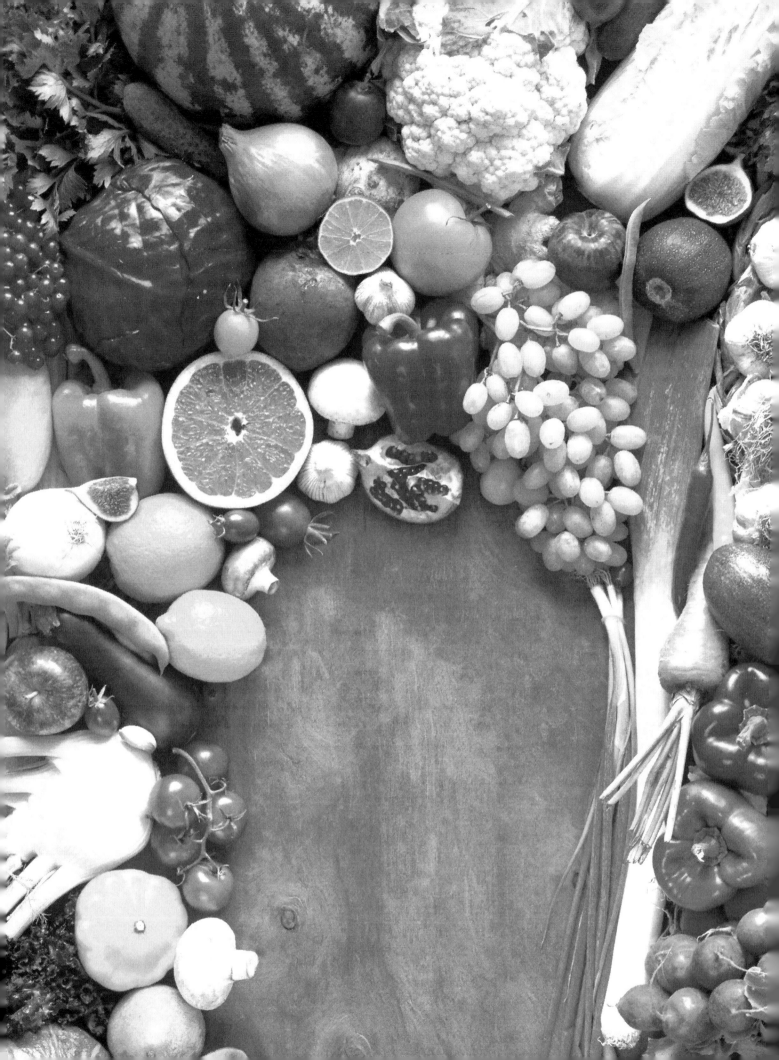

# Contents

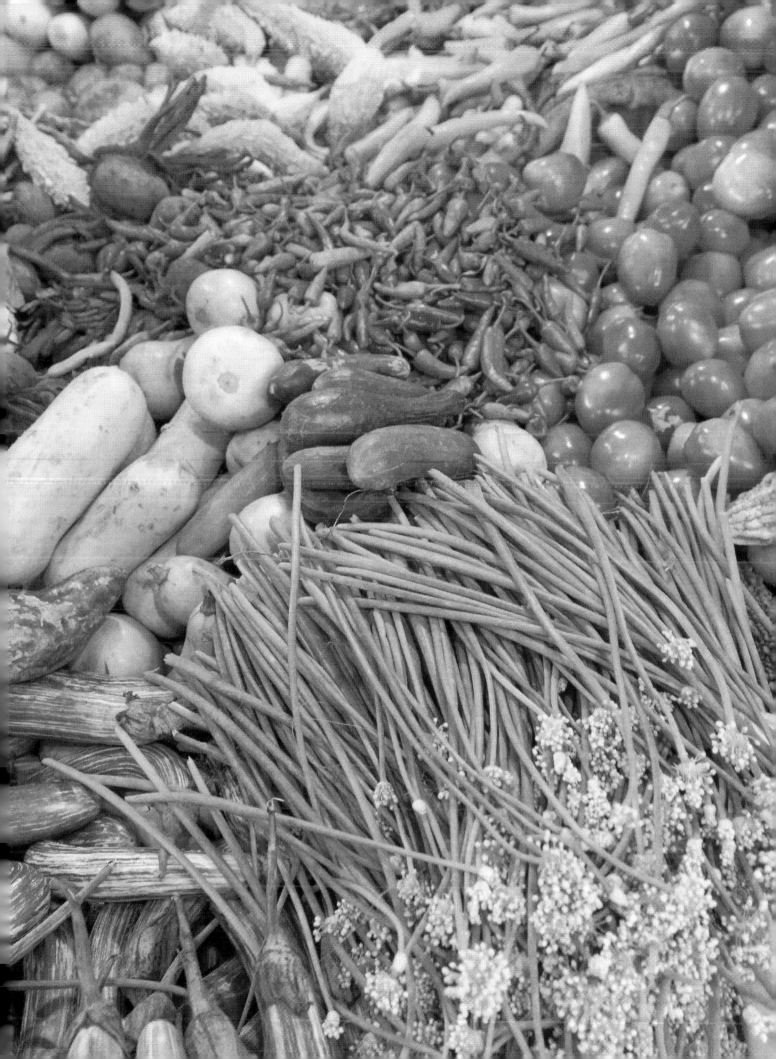

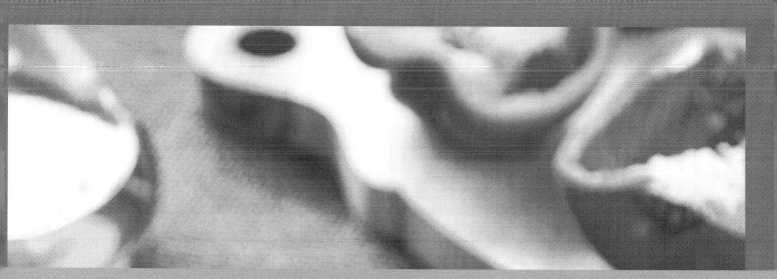

# Introduction

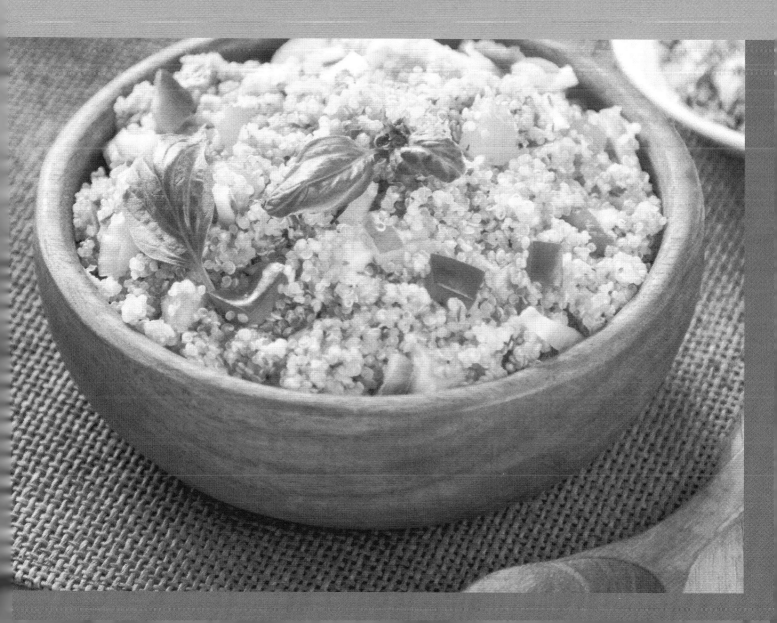

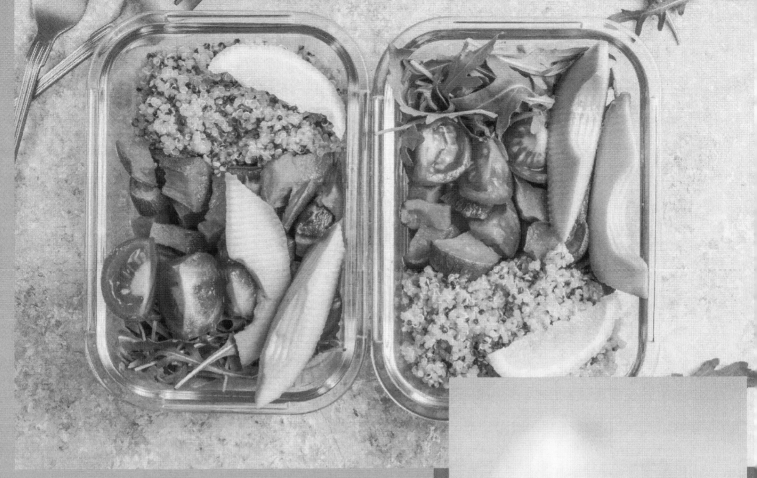

# Introduction

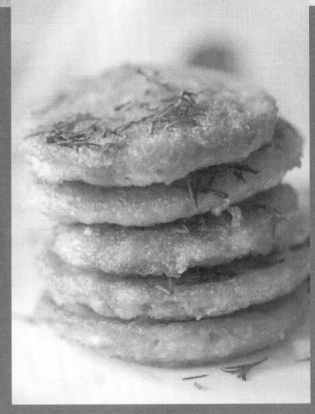

Everything you eat or drink is either alkaline or acidic (or somewhere in between) and will be released into your blood.

If your diet revolves around acidic foods (as most modern diets do), your body is probably overly acidic. Over the years, your bones will become weak, joints and muscles painful, and you will be at a higher risk of developing heart disease, diabetes, kidney disease, and other life-threatening conditions.

This shows that longevity is directly linked to the acid-alkaline balance of your body.

# BACKGROUND

Unfortunately, there is another side to the coin when it comes to eating a plant-based diet. Most people assume that just by being a vegan or vegetarian, you automatically become healthy. This is just a very simplified approach to nutrition.

If you are familiar with Dr. Sebi Alkaline food list, you will notice that many so-called HEALTHY FOODS are missing from the list. The reason is that Dr. Sebi excluded all *hybridized foods* - even if they were alkaline and nutritious, eg potatoes, mint, garlic, parsley, beans, etc.

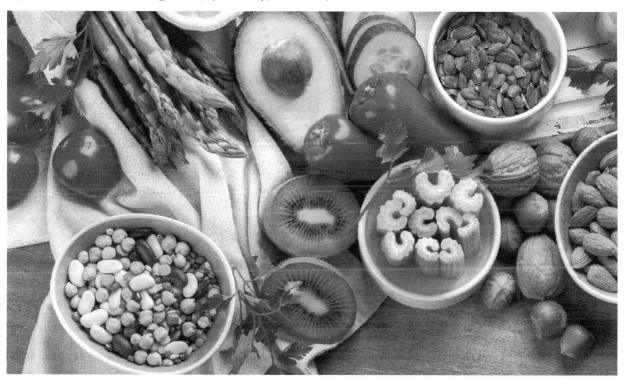

Ingredients that go into a plant-based diet do not have to be healthier than the ingredients of an omnivorous diet. Many of the plant-based foods are not only hybridized but are also genetically modified, eg 98% of Soy. Which makes you wonder how healthy the tofu you eat really is.

Besides, we know that commercially produced fruits and vegetables are heavily treated with pesticides and herbicides. Some fruits are treated once a week for 3-4 months, ie from the moment they flower, until they are picked, eg apples, peaches, etc. That's how you get those perfect-looking fruits.

The trouble is that foods that are not natural, cannot be absorbed properly and can cause disease, so basically eating them is a waste of time and money. Which explains why Dr. Sebi was so passionate about natural foods whose

DNA had not been tampered with.

On top of that, an acidic diet is made even unhealthier by sugar-added foods, additives and preservatives, alcohol, caffeine, etc. So, the problem is not only with a particular food, but with the cumulative effect of a long-term highly acidic diet and lifestyle.

That brings us to the Dr. Sebi Alkaline Diet and Nutritional Guide – the only one and original resource to learn and understand what foods are approved and best for your health as well as foods you should be avoiding no matter the cost.

Also included are best storage and preservation methods for Sebian-approved foods as well as where to source fresh organic foods near you.

# THE ALKALINE-ACID BALANCE

The key principle of two ancient medical systems, Ayurveda and Traditional Chinese Medicine is that health, happiness, and prosperity in life are all based on balance – in diet, behavior, emotions, etc. Although this has for a long time not been taken seriously, mainstream medicine has finally accepted that balance really IS the key to optimal health – physical, mental, and emotional.

When it comes to a diet, it's important to learn how to maintain a balance between acidic and alkaline foods. Although having alkaline blood is better than having acidic blood, if your body becomes too alkaline, you also have a problem. Besides, all your organs and systems are interconnected. So, if you improve one organ or system, functions of other organs related to it will also be improved, e.g., improving cardiovascular health improves the digestive system, the improved nervous system will improve the lymphatic system, etc. And when you improve the overall acid/alkaline balance of the body, you automatically improve the function of all your organs and systems.

So, to maintain health or address a particular health condition, start by improving the pH balance of your blood. This will result in a reduced risk of inflammation, improved bone health, higher energy levels, etc.

However, maintaining healthy blood pH can be tricky. Various organs have different pH and we know that blood pH should range between 7.25 – 7.45. If the pH falls below or rises above this range, you have a problem. Your blood uses a lot of energy to maintain healthy pH levels. This means that if your diet is unhealthy, ie acidic, your body will have to draw the energy it needs not from the foods you eat but from your own reserves. If this goes on for a long time, it may lead to nutrient deficiencies and many health problems.

However, if your pH levels are balanced, your health problems (if you have them) will be resolved naturally because the body is strong enough to heal and repair itself. Besides, a healthy body comes with healthy cells and a strong immune system which is the best protection against infections and chronic conditions, such as cancer or diabetes.

The best and easiest way to maintain a healthy pH level is by adopting an alkaline diet and avoiding stress (because people often eat foods high in sugar when they are trying to distress).

However, eating alkaline foods is not enough. The foods should also be organic because ALL pesticides are very acidic. This is particularly important if you have adopted an alkaline diet to address a particular health problem. Unfortunately, getting organic food is neither easy nor cheap, especially if you have a family to feed. So, if you can't grow your own food, and find buying such foods from specialized shops too expensive, try to buy directly from small farmers who are less likely to use harmful chemicals used for commercial production.

The best source of alkaline foods are fruits and vegetables, however, they come with different pH, ie some are more alkaline than others. Still, you can use this list as a rough guide to foods that will improve your alkaline/acid balance:

- **Fruits**

Apples, avocados, apricots, bananas, cantaloupes, berries, cherries, dates, currants, figs, grapefruits, grapes, guavas, limes, lemons, mangoes, nectarines, melons, oranges, passion fruits, papayas, peaches, persimmons, pineapples, pears, tangerines, raisins.


- **Vegetables**

Bamboo shoots, lima beans, green beans, string beans, beets, sprouts, broccoli, celery, cabbage, cauliflower, chicory, chard, chives, cucumber, collard greens, dandelion greens, dulse, dill, eggplant, escarole, endive, kale, leeks, garlic, legumes, okra, lettuce, onions, parsnip, parsley, sweet potato/yam, white potatoes, bell peppers, pumpkin, rutabaga, radish, watercress, turnips.

### – Nuts

Almonds, walnuts, coconuts

### – Miscel food

Ginger, alfalfa, kelp, clover, sage, mint, green tea, flaxseed, quinoa, pumpkin seeds, all sea veggies

### – Dairy

Vegans don't take dairy but during the transition period, you may take some from time to time as you will probably crave many of the acidic foods you're used to. Although yogurt and kefir are dairy products, they are less acidic than milk or cheese.

*If you are familiar with Dr. Sebi Alkaline Food list, you will notice that many of these foods are missing from Dr. Sebi food list. The reason is that Dr. Sebi excluded all hybridized foods, even if they were alkaline and nutritious, eg potatoes, mint, garlic, parsley, beans, etc.*

Acidifying foods, those that you should stay away from, include meat, dairy, sugar, grains, alcohol, coffee, chocolate, sweets, soda, and processed foods.

To find out your body's pH you can test your urine or saliva. If your urine is too acidic, try adding more veggies to your diet, eg salads, smoothies, soups, etc. If your saliva is too acidic, you probably have a digestion problem. Take digestive enzymes for a couple of days and increase your consumption of greens, eg smoothies, raw salads, steamed veggies, etc.

But what if your urine is too alkaline? This may be the result of some of the supplements you may be taking. High levels of cod liver oil, vitamin D, or magnesium and/or calcium supplements can make your urine too alkaline. Stop taking the supplements for a few days and do the test again. If your urine is still too alkaline, there's probably a digestion issue. Reduce consumption of grains, legumes, and nuts as well as meat and dairy (if you're still taking them). Re-test. Keep on experimenting until your urine tests OK. If your bowels are not working properly, take digestive enzymes for a few days.

Also, in the case of your saliva being too alkaline you need to improve your digestion so you may start taking digestive enzymes. Alternatively, to make your saliva less alkaline, you may take some vitamin C or even some acidic foods. Experiment and keep on re-testing.

Everything you eat or drink is either alkaline or acidic (or somewhere in between) and will be released into your blood. If your diet revolves around acidic foods (as most modern diets do) your body is probably overly acidic. Over the years, your bones will become weak, joints and muscles painful, and you will be at a higher risk of developing heart disease, diabetes, kidney disease, and other life-threatening conditions. This shows that longevity is directly linked to the acid-alkaline balance of your body.

Unfortunately, there is another side to the coin when it comes to eating a plant-based diet. Most people assume that just by being a vegan or vegetarian, you automatically become healthy. This is a very simplified approach to nutrition.

Ingredients that go into a plant-based diet do not have to be healthier than the ingredients of an omnivorous diet. Many of the plant-based foods are not only hybridized but are also genetically modified, eg 98% of soy. Which makes you wonder how healthy the tofu you eat really is.

Besides, we know that commercially produced fruits and vegetables are heavily treated with pesticides and herbicides. Some fruits are treated once a week for 3-4 months, ie from the moment they flower, until they are picked, eg apples, peaches, etc. That's how you get those perfect-looking fruits.

The trouble is that foods that are not natural, cannot be absorbed properly so basically eating them is a waste of time and money. Which explains why Dr. Sebi was so passionate about natural foods whose DNA had not been tampered with.

On top of that, an acidic diet is made even unhealthier by sugar-added foods, alcohol, caffeine, etc. So, the problem is not with any particular food, but with the cumulative effect of a long-term highly acidic diet and lifestyle.

However, even if you just can't give up an unhealthy diet, you can at least try to slightly improve your eating habits.

5 tips on diet improvement:

1. **Have some raw leafy vegetables every day, eg as a salad, smoothie, or a snack**

2. Have some fruit every day, eg as a snack between meals, as a smoothie, or as a fruit salad instead of a dessert.

3. Have green vegetables (cooked or raw) as often as you can, eg broccoli, kale, Brussel sprouts, peppers, etc.

4. Snack on nuts and seeds

5. Have avocado and berries a couple of times a week if you can

## HOW THE BODY INTERACTS WITH ALKALINE FOODS

Your body starts changing from the moment you adopt a vegan and/or raw food diet. The first thing you will notice when you stop taking acidic foods and replace them with electric foods is higher energy levels. The nutrient level of your blood will increase and all your organs and systems will benefit from this change. After a couple of weeks, you will notice major changes in your digestion. You will either have more regular bowel movements or you will experience bloating and flatulence. This is particularly common in those who are not used to fiber-rich foods.

This problem usually resolves itself in a week or so although sometimes, especially if the transition to a new diet was sudden, it may lead to certain digestion problems. On the upside, fiber-rich foods will increase the diversity of bacteria in your gut, which is great because this strengthens your gut and boosts your immune system. On the downside, you may develop an Irritable Bowel Syndrome (IBS). However, how your body reacts to a vegan diet depends partly on whether you're eating processed and refined vegan foods or you're following a whole vegan diet.

After several months on an electric diet, you may experience significant skin improvements and your acne may disappear. However, by now your stores of vitamin D, which you probably got from meat, fish, and dairy, may start dropping. Vitamin D is essential for healthy bones, teeth, and muscles and deficiency is linked with cancer, heart disease, migraines, and depression. The problem is that vitamin D stores last only for about two months. Unless you have regular exposure to sunlight, start eating fortified foods or take supplements.

So, a vegan diet needs to be planned and implemented carefully. If you do, after a few months, your cardiovascular health will improve and this will lower your risk of heart disease, stroke, or diabetes.

However, there is also a paradox, in that the nutrients like iron, zinc, and calcium are reduced on a vegan diet, so the body starts "stealing" them from the intestines. You may consider taking supplements, especially if you don't have time to plan and prepare healthy vegan meals.

After about 6 months on a vegan/raw food diet, your vitamin B12 stores will probably become depleted. This vitamin is essential for healthy blood and nerve cells and can only be found in animal products. Symptoms of B12 deficiency include exhaustion, breathlessness, tingling in the feet or hands poor memory. This can be prevented by taking a supplement. This is very vital because any deficiency will negate the benefits of a vegan diet for heart disease and stroke risk and can cause permanent nerve and brain damage.

There is also your bone health to take into consideration. Minerals from the foods we eat are stored in our bones and up to the age of 30, we can add minerals to this store by eating a nutrient-rich diet. However, after the age of 30, our bones become less and less capable of absorbing these minerals so eating calcium-rich foods becomes very important.

Unless you do, your body will have no other option but to draw the calcium from your skeleton to use for your other organs, which may make your bones very brittle and prone to fractures.

Unfortunately, most vegans have brittle bones and are much more prone to fractures, compared to those on omnivorous diets. Plants high in calcium are kale and broccoli but, unfortunately, plant-based calcium is difficult to absorb so it's best to take supplements.

So although a vegan diet comes with many health benefits, you will only benefit from this way of eating if, by careful planning, you avoid nutrient deficiency.

# THE ALKALINE-ANTI-INFLAMMATORY DIET

One of the trendy ways of boosting your fitness, losing weight, and managing many health problems naturally is to adopt the alkaline diet. Still, most people do not understand the power of nutrition and how much a diet can affect one's health - boosting it or undermining it.

Alkaline diets (there's more than one) are also known as alkaline ash diets and alkaline acid diets. They are very popular among Hollywood celebrities not only because they help you lose weight without actually dieting but also because they are a natural remedy for cancer and arthritis.

So, to improve your overall fitness, health, and lose weight, all you have to do is balance your pH levels. And the higher your pH level (ie the more alkaline your diet is), the easier it becomes to avoid certain chronic and degenerative conditions, such as Alzheimer's and cancer.

Unfortunately, the modern diet revolves around acidic foods, eg meat, wheat, sugar, and processed foods, all of which affect your stomach acid balance. Once broken-down during digestion, these foods leave behind traces of acid ash, which is the main trigger of most gastric diseases.

The alkaline diet revolves around foods that help maintain an optimal pH level in the body. These foods are mainly vegetables, ideally raw.

An alkaline diet is based on two principles:

- You eat as many vegetables as possible (the 80/20 principle)

- You limit or eliminate foods that, once ingested, trigger fermentation

Dr. Sebi took this concept a step further and developed a therapy based on alkaline foods, fasting, and herbal remedies. His alkaline diet protocol and methodology is known for eliminating mucus which are byproducts of toxic waste which has accumulated for long. It does so by alkalizing the blood.

Although this may not be the easiest of the diets, it has helped many people who were written off by conventional medicine. For this diet to be sustainable, it should be consistently followed.

So, to maintain a healthy pH balance, avoid or limit animal protein, wheat, dairy, sugar, and processed foods, as well as coffee, tea, alcohol, and smoking. An easy way to follow an alkaline diet is to ensure that 80% of the food you eat is based on vegetables, fruits, nuts & seeds, and herbs

Dr. Sebi therapy is based on a balanced pH level, cleaning the mucus membranes (in the skin, blood, and lymph), fasting which increases the amount of oxygen in the body, and four gallons of spring water and herbal teas a day to eliminate the accumulated toxins.

According to Dr. Sebi, the root cause of ALL diseases is excess acidity and mucus, by elimination of which, your body automatically starts the self-healing process.

## THE SECRET BEHIND THE ALKALINE DIET

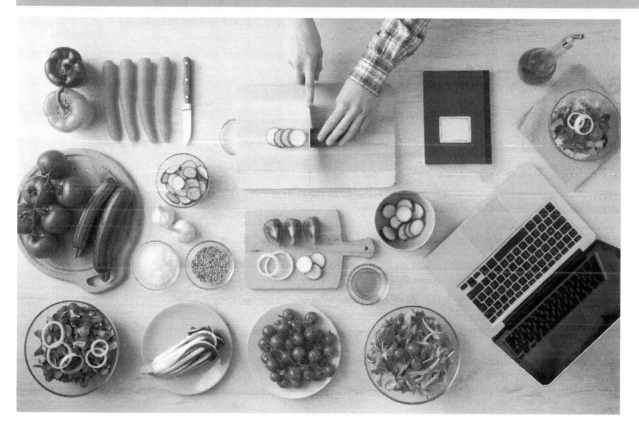

Alkaline diets are about eating in a way that balances your body's pH levels. This balance is necessary for your organs to function well. The main reason that the Western diet is so unhealthy is that it's very acidic, because it's based on meat, sugar, refined wheat, and processed foods. Two reasons excess acidity was much less of a problem in the past are that our diets were then more alkaline and the environment was much less polluted with fewer toxins in the food, water, and air.

The fact that most chronic diseases are diet-related is a double-edged sword. On the one hand, this is good because it means that with a diet change you can easily balance your pH levels. However, bearing in mind that most people eat very unhealthy, slowing down or preventing most chronic diseases such as cardiovascular, diabetes, cancer, autoimmune disorders, and osteoarthritis can be very challenging.

Until about 100 years ago, a typical diet was based on vegetables, a little meat, and whole grains. The modern diet is based on meat, sugar, and dairy.

Fortunately, our body has an amazing self-repair mechanism which, among other things, manages to balance pH levels in our body even when we eat acidic foods.

The pH scale runs from 0 (acidic) to 14 (basic or alkaline), with 7 being neutral.

Ideally, we should try to maintain a pH level of around 7.4. However, not all our organs and fluids require the same acidity level. For example, to be able to break down food, our stomach needs to be very acidic (around 4 pH). Some other organs require even higher acidity, eg duodenum is 7-8.5, small and large intestine 4-7, etc. In other words, all organs that are involved with food processing have high acidity. On the other hand, blood is usually neutral.

Both very high and very low acidity affect our health in a number of ways, so balance is required. But, if this balance is disrupted, you develop either acidosis or alkalosis.

# CHAPTER 1

# THE DR. SEBI NUTRITIONAL GUIDE

Nutrition is a relatively new science and it shouldn't be surprising that we have only relatively recently started paying so much attention to it. Fortunately, we now understand how nutrition affects our physical and mental health and how it can help us avoid disease and heal from one.

Nutrients are ingredients in food essential for overall health. They help us grow, repair body tissue, and build muscle mass. However, even foods known as superfoods cannot provide all the nutrients our body needs to function well. To get all the nutrients we need, you should eat a varied diet.

Things to do if you're serious about your health:

- Find out what your nutritional requirements are
- Figure out where to get them from
- Learn how to combine foods
- Choose the right diet
- Use diet to maintain health or heal
- Eat a variety of foods from each group (ie protein, carbs, fats, vitamins, and minerals)
- Avoid processed foods and sugar
- Get into the habit of reading food labels
- Take supplements, if on a restricted diet

With global health on the decline due to, among other things, unhealthy diets, governments are investing millions of dollars in education and awareness-raising campaigns. One of their better-known efforts is food pyramids. These diagrams represent what type of food you should eat, and how much should certain foods be represented in your diet, ie what should be your staple food and what should be consumed in small quantities or only occasionally.

Food pyramids and the nutrients they claim we need the most of reflect the times we live in as well as the scientific discoveries. They constantly evolve and change and what is considered a healthy diet today is very different from a healthy diet recommended 50 years ago.

Besides, there is no single food pyramid because nutritional guidelines are based on different styles of eating, so we have the Mediterranean Food Pyramid, Vegetarian Food Pyramid, Vegan Food Pyramid, Food Guide Pagoda (China), Ascending Steps to health (France), MyPlate (USA), etc.

But, diets, just like fashion, have trends. The current trend is clean eating and mind/body connection. In other words, a plant-based diet, hydration, and physical activity.

## THE SEBIAN FOOD GROUPS

Dr. Sebi was very particular about food. He insisted that only foods that are 100% alkaline are suitable for a healthy diet. This approach to food developed around the idea that acidity (and mucus that results from it) is the root cause of almost all common health problems. Dr. Sebi was particularly keen on raw and live foods and he believed that cooking destroys food enzymes, making it much less nutritious.

Health experts have argued for years about whether or not stomach acid destroys live food enzymes. Most believed that it did.

However, research by Viktorus Kulvinskas, a prominent expert on nutrition, shows that stomach acid does not destroy the enzymes. It only temporarily deactivates them but they are reactivated when they reach the small intestine, which is more alkaline.

According to Dr. Sebi, all foods can be classified into one of these six groups:

### 1. Live

Live foods look the same way they appear in nature.  These are fruits, vegetables, nuts, seeds, and whole grains. These are believed to be the healthiest food one can eat. The reason they are considered so healthy is that they are high in antioxidants and enzymes, both of which are essential for optimal health. The enzymes promote good digestion by improving the absorption of nutrients and making elimination easy, while antioxidants protect you against disease. This means that a diet based on live foods supports all your organs and functions. As live foods are easily absorbed and thanks to fiber easily eliminated, if you eat them regularly, there will be no toxic waste accumulation.

But, the main benefit of eating live foods is that they are loaded with enzymes that help vitamins and minerals nourish your body. On the other hand, a diet low on live foods and high on dead ones often leads to malnutrition, regardless of how much you eat. A healthy diet high on live foods can replace the supplements. In other words, it's better to assist your digestion with natural fiber and phytonutrients than with enzyme supplements.

To benefit from these nutrients, you should eat food as it was prepared by nature because only in their natural state do foods retain their cellular structure and their original nutritional value. Enzymes are very delicate compounds and are easily destroyed by processing used in commercial food preparation. Consequently, most fruits and veggies are eaten raw, however, some vegetables cannot and should not be eaten raw, eg beans. As for most other live foods, if they are cooked, make sure they still retain their natural color, flavor, and taste.

Besides, some people with weak digestive organs, or the elderly, find it hard to digest raw foods. This doesn't mean they cannot benefit from live foods. Live foods come with many benefits even when steamed, stir-fried, or lightly cooked.

So, regardless of the diet you may be on, even if it includes meat and junk foods, if you make a conscious effort to also include a lot of live foods (in the form of salads or smoothies), you will soon notice, sometimes dramatic improvement of your overall health. Your energy levels will rapidly increase, as will your mental alertness, self-healing power, eyesight, mood, and skin.

## 2. Raw

By raw foods, we usually mean fresh fruits and vegetables, nuts, and seeds. These foods are particularly healthy because they haven't had their enzymes destroyed by heat. Dr.Sebi promoted live and raw foods and he referred to them as "electric foods."

Going raw if you've never eaten this way before is best done gradually, to give your body a chance to adapt to the new diet. While it's true that raw food is more alive, it is also well-known it's more difficult to digest. Besides, as healthy as a raw diet is, some foods contain more nutrients when cooked than when eaten raw, eg Swiss chard, tomato, etc.

The moment you start eating healthy, eg raw, you will start detoxing. However, a sudden detox for which you may be physically or mentally unprepared may be difficult to go through and you may end up developing withdrawal symptoms. Or, the cravings may be so strong they may be impossible to ignore. Once you decide to adopt raw foodism, give yourself at least a month to gradually wean yourself off unhealthy foods by eating more and more raw foods every day.

Help your body adapt to the new diet by preparing yourself for this change. Start by learning as much as you can about raw foodism, as well as about possible side effects and how to deal with them.

While reading up on this diet you will certainly come across views that eating only raw foods is not considered safe.

A raw food diet is a diet based on foods that are never heated over (104-18F or 40-48 C), nor are they pasteurized, or processed in any way. The main reason cooking is discouraged is that it's believed that heat destroys enzymes and nutrients and makes the food less live. However, a lot of debate is going on around this thesis as there are definitely some advantages to cooked foods.

Although cooking does destroy the nutrients, especially vitamins B and C, it also increases the availability of other nutrients and antioxidants, such as lycopene (found in tomatoes) and beta-carotene (found in carrots). This means that some foods actually contain more antioxidants when eaten cooked than raw.

Besides, cooking also helps destroy some harmful compounds found in grains and legumes and also kills bacteria.

Raw foodists believe that there is no need to take any supplements while you're on this diet because raw foods contain all the nutrients your body needs for optimal health.

Foods are you allowed to eat on a raw food diet:

- Sprouts

- Seaweed

- Raw nuts and seeds

- Raw nut butter

- Raw grains and legumes, sprouted or just soaked

- Nut milk

- Fresh vegetables

- Fresh fruits

- Fermented foods

- Dried fruits and veg

- Cold-pressed oil

Foods to avoid on a raw food diet:

- Alcohol

- All baked foods

- All processed foods

- Chips/crackers

- Coffee and tea

- Cooked fruits, vegetables, and grains

- Pasta

- Pasteurized juices and dairy

- Pastries

- Refined oils

- Refined sugars and flour

- Roasted nuts and seeds

Another benefit of a raw food diet is that being high in nutrients and fiber and very low in calories, this diet guarantees a quick weight loss. However, people who are used to a high-calorie diet or who, due to their occupation, need to take a lot of calories, may find it impossible to get all the calories they need from a raw food diet. Besides, cooked foods are not only easily digested, they also make it easier for the body to get calories from them.

Still, a raw food diet comes with many health benefits. It can help you lower blood cholesterol and triglyceride levels, but it also lowers the healthy HDL cholesterol which may lead to a vitamin B12 deficiency. Besides, being on a raw diet for a long time increases your risk of tooth erosion, irregularities in the menstrual cycle (due to low body weight), and low bone mass (due to low calorie and protein intake).

So, in summary, raw foods are super healthy and nutritious, but eating only raw foods for more than a few months at a time could have negative side effects. However, it's perfectly safe to "go raw" for a couple of months twice a year and naturally detox your body.

## 3. Dead

This is the type of food that can't go bad and that is still edible after being on a shelf or in a cupboard for months. Look around your kitchen, it's probably full of such items. Food is killed by being processed, ie treated by heat, (usually very high), packaged, canned, dehydrated, vacuum packed, or ultrapasteurized. Do you know how long-life milk is made? Raw milk is dried at a very high temperature, about 1000 degrees C until all water has evaporated and only the milk powder remains. Then, water is added to that powder and, to turn it into a liquid, a super-fast centrifugal force is used which ensures the cream doesn't separate. As for the nutrients found in natural milk, forget it, nothing can survive such heat and such processing. This is why synthetic nutrients are added to long-life milk. Other long-life foods undergo similar processing. These foods are very dead not just because they lack natural nutrients, they often contain very harmful chemicals.

However, these foods are very convenient and often cheaper than healthy food. They come in the form of TV dinners, snacks, meal replacement bars, crackers, canned and bottled foods, etc. Being high in salt, sugar, color and flavor additives, as well as preservatives, they should be avoided at all costs. They may be convenient in certain situations but should not be part of your regular diet.

## 4. Hybrid

Plants have been hybridized for a very long time. This is done mainly for practical reasons, ie to improve the taste, appearance, or flavor of a fruit, vegetable, or grain. There is no doubt that we have all benefitted from tastier or more palatable foods thanks to hybridization, however looking at this from another angle, this is a typical example of a man playing God and trying to create new species. Dr. Sebi was dead against such foods which is one of the reasons why his food list is so limited. He believed that hybridized foods are unnatural and do not provide nourishment that natural foods do. Unfortunately, almost all the fruits, vegetables, and grains we use today have at some stage been hybridized. While new varieties are being created every year (see Chapter 7),

## 5. Genetically modified (GM)

Species are genetically modified to make them more resistant to disease, to increase yield, or to extend their shelf life. Although not many foods have been genetically modified so far, those that have, ef soybean and corn, are used in the preparation of many other foods, both for human and livestock consumption. This simply means that we have been eating GM foods for many years without realizing it. GM foods are very unhealthy and may lead to lower fertility, allergies, increased appetite and obesity, destruction of biodiversity, etc (see Chapter 7 for more information).

## 6. Drugs

Foods that are regarded as drugs contain substances that, when taken into the body, alter some of the body's functions (physical or psychological). Although we usually think of heroin and cocaine as drugs, drugs also come in other, hidden forms, eg alcohol, caffeine, and tobacco. Both these types of drugs are addictive as all those trying to give up alcohol or smoking can confirm. Taking these legal drugs (ie alcohol, caffeine, cigarettes) not only destroys your own health but also affects the health of those around you.

In the case of smoking, this is self-explanatory as it's well-known that the secondary smoke is as unhealthy as the smoke inhaled directly from cigarettes. So, smokers destroy not only their own health but the health of everyone who has to share their home or work environment (fortunately, most countries have now forbidden smoking in public places).

In the case of alcohol consumption, the psychological and social side effects of being addicted to alcohol or living with someone who is, are well known. Besides, over-consumption can cause a number of serious health conditions from liver cirrhosis to cancer.

Caffeine is probably the least dangerous drug food and it does not affect your environment. Still, it is dehydrating, addictive, sleep-disruptive, and although it has a short-tern pick-me-up effect, it actually contributes to stress and exhaustion. Don't forget that caffeine can also be found in tea and caffeine-rich drinks, eg Coke, Red Bull, etc.

## KEY PRINCIPLES OF DR. SEBI DIET

Dr. Sebi diet and his approach to health and healing are based on three key principles which are all backed by science. They are:

### 1. Dr. Sebi Food List

Dr. Sebi methodology revolves around his alkaline food list. He believed that only natural foods, ie foods created by God, can be nourishing and healing and that all the foods that contribute to mucus formation should be excluded from a healthy diet. Dr. Sebi discouraged the consumption of hybridized foods because he believed they lack the"life force" the body needs to stay healthy. The problem with this is that most of what we eat today has at some stage been crossbred. The hybridization is continuing and our grandparents wouldn't recognize many of the foods we eat today.

The main reason Dr. Sebi hated hybridized foods so much is that he believed that the DNA of a live organism can be tempered with only by God, and not by man. He regarded these foods as artificial and unsuitable for nourishing the body on the cellular level.

### 2. Springwater

Dr. Sebi Alkaline Diet included 4 liters of springwater a day. We all know water is essential for life but as Dr. Sebi methodology revolved around freeing a body from accumulated toxins, he insisted on so much water simply because it helps speed up waste elimination.

This is why Dr. Sebi methodology includes a lot of herbs that act as diuretics and increase urination which naturally flushes out toxins from the body.

Hydration is important even if you eat healthy foods but a standard Western diet that is high on processed and low on live foods requires a lot of water to move the waste from the body. Live foods (fruits and vegetables) have a high water content so those who eat a lot of these foods do not have to take so much water simply because their diets are already high in water.

Unfortunately, most people not only eat unhealthy foods, they also take far too little water. This encourages the accumulation of toxins or their circulation through the body. Uneliminated toxins are either stored in some organs or are reabsorbed by the blood and continue to circulate through your bloodstream over and over again.

So, if you for whatever reason cannot follow a healthy diet and cannot have at least 7 portions of fresh fruits or vegetables a day (every day), at least drink 4 liters of water. Water cannot provide the nutrients that live food can but it will at least help reduce the toxic load.

### 3. No microwaving

Many people, including Dr. Sebi, believe that microwaving is unhealthy and that those who are serious about their health, should never prepare food this way. Of course, thousands of microwave ovens are sold every day because they are very convenient and save a lot of time. However, although a passionate debate is going on around the safety of microwaving, it makes you wonder what sort of force is necessary to cook a meal in ten minutes that would otherwise require hours of cooking.

Dr. Sebi believed that only food cooked on a stove or open fire can be truly healthy and healing.

## DOS AND DONTS

Many regard Dr. Sebi approach to health and diet as very controversial but the fact is that his methodology was based on natural remedies and a diet high in nutritious, energy-promoting, and body-healing foods. The dos and don'ts of Dr. Sebi methodology have a lot to do with one's mindset. In other words, Dr. Sebi diet is more about a lifestyle than just a diet.

### – Commitment

To achieve a goal, any goal you need to commit to it. Commitment to Dr. Sebi lifestyle starts with awareness of how polluted our world has become and how many toxins end up in our body both through an unhealthy diet as well as from environmental toxins. Commit to be toxin-free within six months (or less) and to do everything in your power to eat live and raw foods, organic if possible, and to support your health with medicinal herbs and physical activity.

### – Self-discipline

Following a Dr. Sebi Alkaline diet or a raw food diet for months at a time is not easy especially if you are used to processed foods. So, when tough decisions need to be made, self-discipline and perseverance are crucial. You will certainly face crisis and there will be times when you'll question yourself if the effort is worth it. However, all this can be overcome if you are focused on your final goal – staying healthy or recovering your health after a disease.

### – The belief in the miracle of a plant-based diet

Plants possess the life force that can nourish, heal, calm, or vitalize. It follows that if you adopt a plant-based diet, you stand to benefit from all this.

The magic of plant-based foods is that plants are living organisms who possess both intelligence and energy. They absorb and emit the vibes they collect from their environment and this energy eventually gets transformed into food on your plate or plant medicine.

### – The belief that nature has a cure for all

Some people may find this notion romantic and unrealistic but just think – a lot of medicinal drugs we use today are based on natural herbs. As time goes on and new discoveries are made, we continue to be surprised how healing some herbs really are.

Followers of Ayurveda and Traditional Chinese Medicine are not surprised. They've known about this for more than 5000 years but Westerners were too ignorant and arrogant to accept that it's possible that something as simple as a fruit can be an amazing source of vitamins, that leaves are loaded with antioxidants and fiber, that roots are a source of complex carbohydrates, that flowers are high in phytochemicals, that nuts are such a good source of omega-3 fats, etc. Traditional cultures knew this and survived without mainstream medicine for thousands of years. How sad it is that the developed world is only now catching up.

So, in a nutshell, the recommendations of Dr. Sebi methodology can be summed up as follows:

## DOs:
- Adopt the dr. sebi diet
- Eat only foods that are 100% alkaline
- Gradually start reducing acidic foods in your diet and increasing the

intake of alkaline foods
- Eat only live foods
- Eat raw foods as often as you can
- Cook foods on the stove or over an open fire
- Drink 4 gallons of spring water per day
- Take supplementation if on a restrictive diet
- Detox at least twice a year
- After a cleansing revitalize the body with Dr. Sebi-recommended herbs

**DON'Ts:**
- Don't eat dead, hybridized, or GM foods
- Avoid processed foods
- Substitute acidic foods with alkaline ones: sugar with dried dates, dairy with non-dairy products, refined grains with whole grains, etc.
- Give up or limit smoking and alcohol
- Never use a microwave

# CHAPTER 2
# UNDERSTANDING THE ELECTRIC ALKALINE AND ANTI-INFLAMMATORY DIET

Nutrition is a relatively new science and the concept of electric foods is even more recent. The idea behind this philosophy is that about 90% of what we eat is more or less "dead" and unsuitable for consumption. The modern diet is based on foods that are hybridized (ie most of the staple foods and many fruits and vegetables used today), fortified, genetically modified, heavily processed, or highly toxic (due to pesticides, herbicides, growth hormones, or antibiotics). Is it then surprising that our immunity, overall health, and reproductive health have deteriorated so much that we are plagued with more and more diseases that are difficult to diagnose and even more difficult to cure.

As most of these negative side effects of modern lifestyle and extensive food production have been introduced gradually, over the last hundred years, most people managed to adapt to them - some more than others. However, as the presence of processed foods, GMOs, environmental pollution, and stress have dramatically intensified over the last thirty years, what we are witnessing is a physical and mental decline of the human population on a global scale. Fortunately, these anomalies of modern society could easily be avoided or corrected with a diet change.

And this is where Dr. Sebi philosophy comes in. Dr. Sebi passionately believed that to avoid disease or heal yourself naturally if you are already sick, all you have to do is follow an alkaline diet. But, not just any alkaline diet (there are a few), but a diet based on Dr. Sebi Alkaline Food list. What sets Dr. Sebi alkaline diet apart is that it does not contain any hybridized or GM foods and includes a lot of medicinal herbs and herbal supplements. According to Dr. Sebi, in an alkaline environment, a disease cannot develop let alone thrive and spread.

So, staying healthy is about alkalizing your body. Electric foods can help you do that.

Although conventional medicine is still skeptical about how beneficial an alkaline diet really is, it's not true that the benefits of the alkaline diet are not supported by scientific studies. There are hundreds of research papers published in scientific journals throughout the world which generally agree that an alkaline diet helps reduce morbidity and mortality from chronic disease. We know that certain foods affect the body's pH levels. Good health requires a healthy pH balance within the body. This is necessary because, to function properly, organs and fluids need a balanced pH level.

To understand the importance of an alkaline diet, you have to know why our modern diet is so acidic. Ever since we started practicing agriculture and adopted a settled lifestyle, our diet has been steadily changing. This happened about 10,000 years ago and this period is known as the Agricultural Revolution. Although this seems like a very long time, in an evolutionary sense, this is like something that happened just a few minutes ago. So, until about 200 years ago, our diet wasn't that bad. Although many of the foods were hybridized, our lifestyle was still not as sedentary as it is today, the environment contained much fewer toxins than it does today, and our diet did not contain processed foods. We ate mainly natural carbs, vegetables, and only occasionally, meat. The main sources of sugar were fruits. Foods were minimally processed. Then, the Industrial Revolution changed everything. Ever since, our diet has contained more and more refined grains, unhealthy fats, commercially processed meats and sugar. It also became increasingly rich in inflammatory foods.

As most of the chronic diseases of civilization are diet-related, it's obvious that something is very wrong with our eating habits. The life-threatening diseases plaguing the modern world, which can all be reversed with a healthy diet are obesity, diabetes, cardiovascular disease, cancer, autoimmune disorders, depression, amongst others. Compared to what we eat today, the diet of 200 or more years ago was very alkaline. It was based on whole grains, little or no meat, and naturally grown organic fruits and vegetables. Combined, these foods produced a "net alkaline effect."

# pH scale

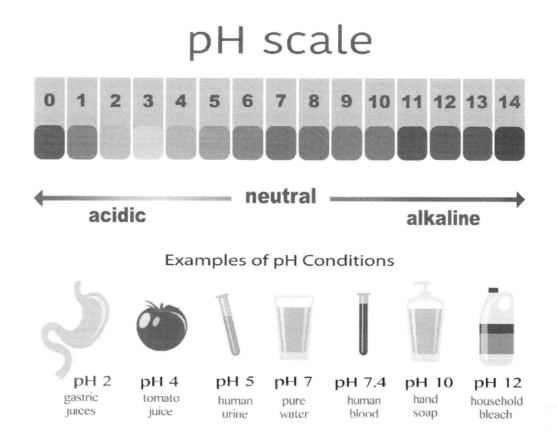

The PH scale depicting acidity and alkalinity

The human body is an amazing organism and the reason we have as a species survived for so long is that our body has means of self-repair. This includes maintaining good pH levels regardless of what we eat. The pH scale runs from 0 to 14. While 0 is acidic, 14 is alkaline or basic; and the midpoint, 7 is neutral. Ideally, pure water is on a scale of pH 7.

Ideally, we should try to maintain a pH level of around 7.4. However, not all our organs and fluids require the same acidity level. For example, to be able to break down food, our stomach needs to be acidic (around 4 pH). Some other organs require even higher acidity, e.g. duodenum is 7-8.5, small and large intestine 4-7, etc. So, organs that are involved with food processing have high acidity. On the other hand, blood is usually neutral. When the pH level of a particular organ or system becomes too high or too low, this affects our health in many ways. For instance, the inside of your stomach is lined with a thick layer of mucus that protects it from being destroyed by your stomach's natural acidity. On the other hand, the small intestine has alkaline bile released into it which offers protection from the stomach acidity.

Proper pH is essential for good health and an extreme imbalance (either too much or not enough of acidity) can be fatal. In the absence of balance, you develop either acidosis or alkalosis. Acidosis is characterized by high acidity. There are several different types of acidosis: respiratory, metabolic, renal (kidneys), and lactic acidosis. Symptoms include fatigue, lethargy, confusion, and shortness of breath. Furthermore, metabolic acidosis is the commonly associated with the alkaline diet, but this condition can also be the result of kidney disease or dehydration. Besides, this type of acidosis increases your risk of developing cardiovascular disease, diabetes, insulin resistance, and kidney stones. Diet-induced metabolic acidosis is the consequence of eating too much meat, and not enough fruits and vegetables.

On the other hand, alkalosis is also a potentially dangerous health condition. It occurs when blood or bodily fluids become EXTREMELY alkaline. It's a condition that can be caused by low oxygen levels, a sudden loss of electrolytes or lung or liver disease. Symptoms include confusion, lightheadedness, and muscle spasm, seizure, tingling in the extremities and face, and respiratory problems.

## DOES THE ALKALINE DIET WORK?

An alkaline diet is based on the assumption that certain foods promote either alkalinity or acidity in the body. However, mainstream science does not support this theory. Very acidic foods indeed cause kidneys to excrete more acid, but having acidic urine doesn't have to mean that your overall pH levels are high. Measuring your acidity through urine is not a reliable method of checking your pH levels because it does not show how acidic your whole body is. Different fluids in our body require different pH levels to function properly. For example, an average pH for urine is from 4.6 to 8, while blood pH it's about 7.4.

Under normal circumstances, our body is perfectly capable of getting rid of excess acid. Its secret weapons against acidosis are kidneys and lungs. The kidneys maintain a healthy pH level by removing excess acid via urine. However, when kidneys are not working well, excretion of urine can slow down or stop. This is a potentially very dangerous situation because it means that urine will start accumulating in the body, making it even more acidic. This condition usually gets worse with age, as kidney functions slowly but steadily decrease. Another organ crucial for maintaining balanced pH levels is the lungs. Carbon dioxide which is a byproduct of cell metabolism creates acidity in the blood. If your lungs work well, they'll be able to maintain a balanced pH level by regulating respiratory functions as necessary.

The purpose of an alkaline diet is to help you maintain healthy pH levels within all your organs. However, people follow this diet for many other reasons, e.g. to lose weight, to have more energy, to avoid or reverse diabetes, etc. To know if a specific diet "works" or not, you have to be clear why you are on that diet. Only when you have a goal, will you be able to determine whether the diet works or not. Your goal may be to lose weight, build muscle, detox your body, etc. and only by occasionally revisiting your goals will you be able to decide if you've been successful or not.

Although the alkaline diet is somewhat limiting because it excludes many nutritious foods, it is generally a very healthy diet simply because it revolves around healthy foods, i.e. potassium-rich fruits and vegetables. This is why many nutritionists believe that the reason this diet is so healthy may have more to do with the type of foods it is based on, than with the balanced pH levels.

## WHAT ARE ELECTRIC ALKALINE FOODS?

Electric food is food that is natural and live, which is just what your body needs to feel alive. Unfortunately, about 80% of foods in a typical Western diet are not electric. On top of that, over 90% of those foods are hybrids that are usually highly acidic and that prevent the absorption of nutrients on a cellular level. Obesity is a growing problem especially in the developed world, mainly because, despite all the food you eat, if it lacks nutrients, your body will starve on a cellular level. And when you are starving, you will want to eat but as the food you eat is usually just empty calories and your body is not really nourished, it will continue to be hungry, and you will continue to eat, and so the vicious circle continues.

Generally speaking, a modern diet is very low in nutrients. Even if you are one of those people who read the labels to check that the food you buy contains sufficient nutrition, what you probably don't realize is that those are synthetic nutrients that have been added to already dead food. Such food, being dead, cannot be properly absorbed and processed by the body.

So, it's not enough to take a certain amount of nutrients. The nutrients have to be taken in a form that your body can process and absorb. Which is not what a modern diet can do for you. On the contrary, it was created (intentionally or out of ignorance) to set us up for disease, low immunity, and addiction to antibiotics, sedatives, or sleeping pills.

Fortunately, you can avoid this trap by adopting an electric diet. How do you start?

### – Adopt an electric lifestyle

Electric foods should become a part of your every meal every day for the rest of your life. So, this is more than just a diet. To maintain health or recover from a disease with the help of electric foods, approach an electric diet as a lifestyle.

### – Education

Learn which foods you need to avoid and which to introduce or eat more of. If you've lived on a very acidic diet so far, you will have to introduce these changes gradually.

### – Cleanse

To give yourself a new lease on life (which you will, with this diet) start by cleansing your body from the accumulated toxins, mucus, and fat. After the cleanse revitalize your body with Dr. Sebi revitalizing herbs.

### – Commitment

Commit to rid yourself of unhealthy habits and addictions

As part of your new lifestyle, you will need to download a list of alkaline foods from the Internet. Don't be surprised if you come across different lists. Although all fruits and vegetables are alkaline, their pH levels vary. For a start, avoid acidic foods but during the transition period, you may eat some foods that are moderately acidic (eg dairy is acidic but yogurt is much less acidic than milk or cheese). You may find that an alkaline diet is more expensive than an ordinary diet (based on processed foods), so work out how to live on a vegan diet on a budget.

Also, print out a list of common hybrid foods and take it with you when you go shopping. Some of them are easy to recognize:

- They lack seeds (eg seedless grapes, watermelon, apples, grapes, tangerines, etc).
- They may have an unusual color (eg yellow watermelon, yellow cherry

tomatoes, black tomatoes, etc).

- Their name is an obvious combination of two plants, eg kalettes (Brussel sprouts and kale), peacotum (peach, apricot, and plum), etc.

3 main reasons you should avoid hybrids whenever you can:

1. They are high in sugar and starch. This sugar cannot be absorbed or used by the pancreas and liver.

2. Most of them don't have a proper mineral balance which, over time, may lead to nutrient imbalance.

3. Some hybrid foods can make Candida worse.

The common hybrid foods include carrots, corn, beets, celery, potatoes, cauliflower, rice, cashews, oats, soy, wheat, legumes, echinacea, garlic, ginseng, chamomile, etc (see Chapter 7 for a full list).

# SCIENCE BEHIND FOOD ELECTRICITY

Dr. Sebi referred to live and raw foods as electric foods. However, it wasn't only Dr. Sebi's view. Although the health benefits of vegan and raw diets were for a long time disapproved by mainstream science, things have, fortunately, changed.

However, not all vegan diets are created equal. They need to be carefully planned so you continue to get sufficient essential acids, vitamin B12, and essential minerals. It's absolutely crucial to stay away from most ready-made vegan meals as they are simply a vegan version of processed foods.

6 science-based health benefits of a vegan and a raw food diet:

### 1. It's loaded with nutrients

Vegan diets are based on fruits and vegetables and raw food diets are based on raw fruit and vegetables. Both these diets are high in fiber, vitamins, minerals, and antioxidants. They are also a significant source of potassium, magnesium, folate, and vitamins A, C, and E.

### 2. It helps with weight management

Vegans are rarely overweight and if they eat natural vegan foods, they simply cannot be. Many people adopt a vegan diet in an attempt to lose weight naturally.

### 3. It lowers blood sugar levels and improves kidney function

A vegan diet is a natural remedy for high blood sugar levels. Besides, diabetics who substitute meat for plant protein can easily reduce the risk of kidney disease.

### 4. Protects against some types of cancer

Studies suggest that eating fresh fruit and vegetables every day significantly lowers your risk of cancer. Besides, just avoiding animal products, even if you don't eat a lot of fruit and veg, is enough to reduce the risk of prostate, breast, and colon cancers.

### 5. Lowers the risk of heart disease

Vegans rarely have high blood pressure and one of the ways of reducing yours is to adopt a vegan diet. A vegan diet will quickly reduce both blood sugar and bad cholesterol levels.

### 6. Reduces arthritic pains

Numerous reports suggest that people struggling with arthritis would greatly benefit from an alkaline vegan diet. Consistent use of fruits and vegetables, especially raw ones, can successfully reduce pain, joint swelling, and morning stiffness, as well as provide more energy and a better mood (due to the absence of pain).

# DR. SEBI APPROVED ALKALINE & ANTI-INFLAMMATORY FOODS

Based on everything said so far, determining electric foods is about approaching your diet strategically. From now on, your shopping list needs to focus on live and/or raw foods. Ideally, they should be organically-grown, but if this is not possible, at least make sure you stay away from hybridized and GM foods. Print out a list of common hybridized foods (see Chapter 7 for more details) or simply eat according to the attached Dr. Sebi Alkaline Food List.

The list is pretty restrictive and living on it month after month may not be easy. Some of the foods may not be available where you live or may not be affordable if you have a family to feed. In that case, simply eat as many foods from this list as you can while trying to avoid unhealthy foods as much as possible.

So, although it's easy to know what electric foods are, incorporating them into your diet is more difficult. Depending on what kind of vegan diet you follow, eg ordinary vegan diet, raw food vegan diet, or Dr. Sebi alkaline diet, you should create a list of foods your diet should consist of. If this is a problem, follow the 80/20 principle, ie if you eat healthy 80% of the time, it's perfectly OK to eat unhealthy for the remaining 20%. It's not ideal but it's better than nothing. Remember that, to avoid nutrient deficiency, a long-term vegan needs to take certain supplements.

## Dr. Sebi-approved foods include:

VEGETABLES:

1. Amaranth
2. Arame
3. Avocado
4. Bell Pepper
5. Chayote
6. Cherry and Plum Tomato
7. Cucumber
8. Dandelion Greens
9. Dulse
10. Garbanzo Beans
11. Hijiki

12. Izote flower and leaf
13. Kale
14. Lettuce except for iceberg
15. Mushrooms except for Shitake
16. Nopales
17. Nori
18. Okra
19. Olives
20. Onions
21. Purslane Verdolaga
22. Sea Vegetables
23. Squash
24. Tomatillo
25. Turnip Greens
26. Wakame
27. Watercress
28. Wild Arugula
29. Zucchini

## FRUITS:

1. Apples
2. Bananas
3. Berries
4. Cantaloupe
5. Cherries
6. Currants
7. Dates
8. Figs
9. Grapes
10. Limes
11. Mango
12. Melons
13. Orange
14. Papayas
15. Peaches
16. Pears
17. Plums
18. Prickly Pear
19. Prunes
20. Raisins
21. Soft Jelly Coconuts
22. Soursops

23.     Tamarind

## SPICES AND SEASONING:

1. Achiote
2. Basil
3. Bay Leaf
4. Cayenne
5. Cloves
6. Dill
7. Habanero
8. Onion Powder
9. Oregano
10.     Powdered Granulated Seaweed
11.     Pure Sea Salt
12.     Sage
13.     Savory
14.     Sweet Basil
15.     Tarragon
16.     Thyme

## GRAINS:

1. Amaranth
2. Fonio
3. Kamut
4. Quinoa
5. Rye
6. Spelt
7. Tef
8. Wild Rice

## NUTS AND SEEDS:

- Brazil Nuts (Added)
- Hempseed
- Sesame Seeds
- Walnuts
- Sesame "Tahini" Butter

- Pine Nuts

## SUGARS AND SWEETENERS:

1. Date Sugar from dried dates
2. 100% Pure Agave Syrup from cactus

## OILS

- Olive oil
- Hemp seed oil
- Coconut oil
- Sesame oil (unrefined)
- Grapeseed oil
- Avocado oil

# SUPPOSEDLY "HEALTHY" FOODS THAT ARE NOT SEBI-APPROVED

The Dr. Sebi alkaline diet is more than just an alkaline diet. Many foods that are known to be very healthy, and that vegans consume regularly, are not approved by Dr. Sebi. The exclusion is usually based on two facts:

### 1. The foods are not 100% alkaline

Although a plant-based diet is usually considered alkaline, the acidity level of fruits and vegetables can vary greatly. While most vegetables are alkaline (which is why they are considered more important in a diet than fruits), many fruits are naturally acidic (e.g., apples and berries), although this often depends on a variety (e.g., there are sour and sweet apples).

### 2. The foods are hybridized

When it comes to how natural certain foods are, things are a bit complicating. Agriculture is over 10,000 years old and during that time, most of the foods that were initially collected from the wild, have been hybridized – some more than others.

Everything we eat today originated in the wild and was, at some stage, cross-bred either to improve the taste (e.g., make it less sour), increase the size (e.g., wild apples are the size of walnuts), or make the skin thinner and more palatable (e.g., ancient types of beans were so high in fiber that although they were not poisonous, they were quite toxic).

Berries are some of the healthiest foods there are, and they can still be found growing wild in rural regions (e.g., strawberries, raspberries, blackberries, and blueberries) but their fruit is the size of a pea. When you compare such berries to the berries available in the shops, you realize that everything, including Dr. Sebi-approved foods, is actually hybridized.

# ACIDIC VS ALKALINE

Acidic foods have a pH of 4.6 or lower. Acidity in foods may be natural (e.g., most fruits) or added (e.g., pickled veggies). Acid is essential for preventing bacterial growth which is why it has to be added to vegetables you want to preserve by pickling. The more alkaline a vegetable, the more acid you have to add, and vice versa. Food acidity can be increased by the addition of lemon juice, citric acid, or vinegar. Low-acid foods (e.g., oranges) have a pH of 4.6 to 6.9, while alkaline foods (e.g., leafy greens) have a pH of 7.0 or greater.

So, eating only alkaline foods would limit your food choice to such an extent that you would have to eat only leafy greens which would not only be boring but would also not be very healthy. This is why low-acid foods have to be added even to an alkaline diet. Besides, pH varies between varieties, e.g., tomatoes and apples can be very sweet or rather sour, etc. What complicates things even more, is that food charts are based on different criteria which is why you often find conflicting information regarding certain foods. This is also the case with acid/alkaline food charts. This disparity is largely due to how the acid load is calculated because there are more ways than one.

Some classifications are done based on calculations of acidity BEFORE the food is consumed, while others calculate the acidity AFTER the food has been consumed. This explains why some foods that are believed to be alkaline are actually acid-causing. For example, bananas are high in the alkaline mineral potassium, however, they also contain 25% sugar. This makes them very acidifying once they reach your stomach.

All this sounds very complicating but it shouldn't be. It's impossible to eat healthy if you eat strictly alkaline foods but by sticking to a plant-based diet, particularly an alkaline vegan diet, you will easily alkalize your body and get rid of mucus and toxins. An alkaline diet will also help resolve many of your health conditions.

The same applies to acidity. Most fruits are more or less acidic, including those approved by Dr. Sebi. However, some are much more acidic than others so it is these that you should avoid. The reason fruits are acidic is because they are high in sugar. This is why many weight-loss diets recommend you keep fruit consumption to a minimum although this doesn't mean you shouldn't eat them because they are the best source of vitamins and many antioxidants. However, if you are trying to lower the acidic load in your body, don't take more than one fruit a day, e.g., an apple, a bunch of grapes, a plateful of berries, a few plums, etc.

It's interesting that key limes have almost no sugar which is why they taste sour. However, being high in minerals, when ingested, they have an alkaline effect on the body. The same applies to fermented foods, which are normally acid-forming but once they get into your body, they become alkaline.

Still, certain foods that we think of as very healthy, should not be a part of Dr.

Sebi-alkaline diet. The reasons for the exclusion vary but they usually revolve around the following:

<u>5 reasons Dr. Sebi didn't approve many healthy foods:</u>

### 1. *They are very acidic*

A plant-based diet becomes acidic if you take a lot of sugar, eg honey, fruits, etc.

### 2. *They are high in sugar*

Most fruits are high in sugar, especially dried fruits.

### 3. *They can only be raised with a lot of chemical fertilizers*

Some foods are laden with pesticides so much that they are only safe to eat if they are organically grown. This applies particularly to celery stalks, strawberries, and peaches.

### 4. *They are GMO-produced*

This applies to soy and corn, as well to all products that contain soy and corn derivates (eg oil, syrup, etc). As over 90% of all soy and corn produced in the US are genetically modified, only organically grown soy and corn are safe to eat.

### 5. *They are over hybridized*

Although most of what we eat has been hybridized, it has been suggested that it would be best to avoid foods that our grandparents would not recognize.

## THE FOODS NOT APPROVED BY DR. SEBI INCLUDE:

### 1. Lemon

Although very sour, lemon becomes alkaline once ingested. However, lemons as we know them today are hybridized fruit.

### 2. Garlic

Hybridized.

### 3. Ginger

The problems may arise only due to overconsumption. Ginger may interact with certain medications so if you take a lot of ginger and are on chronic medication, talk to your doctor. Besides, taking too much ginger may cause diarrhea and heart conditions, as well as increase the risk of miscarriage. It may also significantly lower your blood pressure.

### 4. Beets

Beets are moderately alkaline but being high in oxalate so too much beetroot juice may increase the risk of developing kidney stones, stomach upsets, or dips in blood pressure.

### 5. Carrots

As a hybridized vegetable, it should not be included in Dr. Sebi diet.

### 6. Corn

Although it does have some health benefits, corn has been hybridized over and over again for hundreds of years. Besides, most of the corn produced in the US is genetically modified.

### 7. Potatoes

After years of eating a lot of potatoes or eating them often, you may develop stomach upsets, eg bloating, constipation, or pain. Like all rapidly digesting carbohydrates, potatoes may also lead to high blood pressure or insulin resistance, ie to Type 2 diabetes.

### 8. Turmeric

Although very healthy and a part of many Ayurvedic therapies, not everyone responds well to this herb. In some people, turmeric may cause bleeding that will not stop, high blood sugar (i.e., increased thirst, increased urination, dry mouth, headache, dizziness, blurred vision, etc.). If you're not used to this herb and start taking a lot of it for its cancer- and inflammation-fighting properties, and experience any of these side effects, stop immediately. However, please note that these side effects can only happen with long-term overconsumption.

### 9. Broccoli

Hybridized.

### 10.      Honey

Animal based. Very acidic.

## 11.    Soy

There is so much conflicting information on soy, that even scientists cannot agree on how healthy or not it is. Soybeans are very high in phytic acid and this may cause mineral deficiencies. Besides, some people not only eat a lot of soy and soy products but most of these products are processed foods. Besides, over 90% of all soy produced in the US is genetically modified which makes soy consumption risky. However, fermented soy products have a lower content of phytic acid and saponin and are therefore safe to eat (provided they are organically grown). Fermented soy products are also a great source of probiotics.

## 12.    Beans

All beans except Garbanzo, are acidic veggies.

## 13.    Spinach

Being high in oxalate, spinach may cause certain intestinal problems. If you eat too much spinach, this can interfere with your body's ability to absorb some important minerals, eg calcium, magnesium, zinc, etc. Besides, spinach is high in fiber so overconsumption often leads to bloating, stomach cramps, intestinal gas, etc. So, you shouldn't take more than one cup of cooked spinach a day.

## 14.    Celery stalks

Celery stalks are probably the most popular vegetable for weight management diets. The main side effect of this vegetable are an allergic reaction, cystic acne, and bloating. However, the production of celery stalks requires a lot of pesticides and it is believed to have the highest content of pesticides of all the fruits and vegetables. Therefore, avoid it unless you can get organically grown ones.

## 15.    Some Oranges

Although an excellent source of vitamin C, having too many oranges day after day may lead to osteoporosis. This happens because when you eat a lot of oranges, more calcium is released from your body that your body can create. This, in turn, weakens your bones and makes you vulnerable to osteoporosis. Besides, oranges contain a lot of sugar which is acid-producing.

## 16.    Some Dried fruits

Highly acidic due to a very high sugar content

### 17.     Some Apples

Moderately acidic, depending on the variety.

### 18.     Apricot

Moderately acidic

### 19.     Banana (Except Burro or Baby bananas)

Moderately acidic

### 20.     Berries

Moderately acidic

### 21.     Grapes

Moderately acidic

### 22.     Mango

Moderately acidic

### 23.     Peach

Moderately acidic

### 24.     Papaya

Moderately acidic

### 25.     Pineapple

Dr. Sebi Alkaline and Anti-inflammatory Diet for Beginners

## HYBRIDIZED VS NATURAL FOODS

When it comes to hybridized fruits and vegetables, Dr. Sebi's recommendations were very clear – you should stay away from these whenever possible. Unfortunately, it is easier said than done. Although some vegetables, e.g., plumcot and broccoflower are obviously a recent hybrid, almost all the fruits and veggies we eat today (including those approved of by Dr. Sebi) were at some stage hybridized (see chapter 7 for more details).

For example, apple or plum (both of which are approved by Dr. Sebi), come from wild apple and wild plum that still exist today but that are much smaller, very sour, and have thicker skin than the fruits available in shops. The same applies to garlic, onions, many types of green leafy vegetables from which, after years of cross-breeding, we managed to get kale, spinach, Swiss chard, broccoli, etc.

So, is it possible to follow a diet based on natural and alkaline foods only? Not really, unless you're prepared to start foraging for food.

Still, following an alkaline diet is the easiest and cheapest way of preventing disease or recovering from one.

## DEAD, HYBRID, AND GMO FOODS

An alkaline diet is considered one of the healthiest diets one can follow. However, although fruits and vegetables are alkaline foods, some are more alkaline than others. This is why Dr. Sebi Alkaline Diet is different from most other alkaline diets. Dr. Sebi food list contains only foods that are 100% alkaline and that are not hybridized. For obvious reasons, the choice of foods allowed on this diet is rather limited so combining them to create balanced, varied meals takes time.

## DEAD FOODS

The reason some foods are called "dead foods" is that they can't go bad – they've already been killed. All foods that can remain safe to eat even if kept out of a fridge or deep-freeze for weeks or months, can safely be called dead.

What these foods have in common is that they are highly processed, contain no fiber, have no nutritional value, and often have synthetic nutrients added to them. On top of that, they always contain food preservatives. Typical examples are crackers, meal replacement bars, fruit snacks, flavored beverages, margarine, etc. Sadly, these foods are very popular partly because they are tasty and convenient, and partly because of the aggressive marketing campaigns that claim they are just what you need to stay healthy. Actually, the toxins these foods contain is the LAST thing you need to put into your body that is already compromised by a polluted environment and unhealthy lifestyle. Besides, long-term consumption of dead foods can wreak havoc in your digestive tract by killing off millions of friendly bacteria that boost your immune system and provide a natural defense against pathogens.

Living on a diet low in nutrients and high in empty calories, synthetic additives, and harmful preservatives is very stressful to the body and it will, sooner or later, become plagued with inflammatory conditions, aches and pains, chronic fatigue, brain fog, poor sleep, weight gain, etc.

Unfortunately, long-term nutrient deficiency can also lead to serious health conditions, e.g., heart disease, diabetes, cancer, high blood pressure, high blood sugar levels, arthritis, etc.

Simple advice – stay away from these foods.

## HYBRID FOODS

Cross-pollination of plants is not a 20th-century invention. It has been practiced for hundreds of years usually as an attempt to develop a new species of plant that will have traits of both plants used in cross-pollination.

Please note that hybridization is very different from Genetically Modified Organisms (GMOs). Hybridized plants use the natural traits of the plants, while GMO adds certain traits to a plant that are not natural to that plant.

Plant hybridization is used to create flowers of different colors, fruit and vegetables that taste better or have thinner skin, etc. Besides, we know that hybridized varieties last much longer so many plants are hybridized simply extend their shelf life. This is particularly common with fruits and vegetables that quickly go off, e.g., raspberries or tomatoes. Another reason for hybridization is that hybridized foods are often more nutritious than the original plants, or are easier to digest.

Most of the fruits and vegetable available today have, at some stage, been hybridized, however new hybridized plants (fruits, vegetables, flowers, and herbs) appear all the time, eg

- Broccolini (broccoli and Chinese cabbage)
- Brokali (broccoli and kale)
- Kalettes (Brussel sprouts and kale)
- Angello (seedless pepper)
- Black galaxy tomato (blueberry and tomato)
- Pluerry (plum and cherry)
- Peacharine (peach and nectarine)
- Plumcot (plum and apricot)
- Peacotum (peach, apricot, and plum)
- Blood lime (red finger lime and Ellendale Mandarin)
- Limequat (key lime and kumquat)
- Pineberry (wild South American strawberry and the North American strawberry)
- Tayberry (blackberry and red raspberry)
- Longaberry (blackberry and red raspberry)
- Tangelo (tangerine and pomelo or grapefruit)
- Broccoflower (broccoli and cauliflower): 2 varieties Romanesco and Green Cauliflower

# GENETICALLY MODIFIED FOODS (GMO)

Genetical modification is the process of altering the genes of living things so that new organisms have, or lack, certain qualities. These new organisms are called genetically modified organisms (GMOs).

In other words, GMOs have their DNA altered in a way that could never have happed by natural reproduction.

GM foods are assessed for safety by checking if they contain toxic ingredients, what their nutritional value is, and whether they could cause allergic reactions. GMO producers claim that GM foods are made available only after it's determined they do not represent a threat to human health. Unfortunately, the situation is not as simple as that

In the EU, GM foods must be labeled, but in the USA and Canada, such foods are not labeled. GM foods come mainly as flour and oil made from soy and corn. These products would be easy to avoid but unfortunately, they are used in the production of many other foods, e.g., cheese is produced with GM enzymes; meat, dairy, and eggs come from animals that are fed GM animal feed, etc. None of these products are labeled.

Producers of GM foods claim that such foods come with a number of benefits, e.g.

## – Health

GM technologies can improve the nutritional value of food. The best-known example is the "golden rice" which is rice loaded with provitamin A that our bodies can convert into vitamin A. GMO producers claim this can prevent vitamin A deficiency. Other "enriched" staple foods include potato (GM potato is enriched with proteins) and cassava (GM cassava provides a day's nutrition in a single meal). Producers also claim that the production of GM foods reduces the need to have the workers exposed to harmful pesticides. Besides these foods have a much longer shelf life.

Plants can even be modified to contain protein, vaccines, and other pharmaceutical products, e.g., tobacco plants can be modified to produce therapeutic antibodies.

## – Economic

GM crops are resistant to insects, disease, and climate change which makes crop management easier and provides increased yield, ie increased income for farmers. **However, the World Health Organization (WHO) suggests that "experimenting with genes can cause undesirable developmental and physiological effects and that GMOs carry significant risk for human health".**

While in the EU, GM foods are treated as "new food" and are subject to extensive evaluations by the European Food Safety, in the US, these foods have been used for human consumption for decades. Some have proven deadly and had to be withdrawn from shops but only after a number of people died as a consequence of eating them (in the 1960s a GM potato was used to make chips but after a number of deaths, had to be withdrawn). This clearly shows that in the US at least, GM foods are deemed "safe" until proven otherwise. And the companies producing these foods still claim they are thoroughly checked for any toxic ingredients and allergens.

A recently released US study confirms that GMOs should not have been allowed on the market until more research into their safety had been done. It is no longer a secret that GM foods are directly linked to the fast deteriorating physical and mental health of the US population and that they are directly linked to 22 serious diseases.

If GM foods cannot be banned, they should at least be labeled so people can make an educated decision whether to buy such foods or not. The only thing that US citizens can do at the moment to protect themselves from GMOs is to buy organic, look for non-GMO seal, and avoid crops where GMOs are common (e.g., soy, corn, etc.).

Besides, with more and more GM crops being used worldwide, there is a very real danger that a contagious virus strain might rapidly spread to other crops. Experiments have shown that GM genes are easily transferred to weeds that grow around crops. This is potentially very dangerous as such weeds could become a "pool" of such viruses even if GM crops are no longer produced. What's particularly worrying is that once genes spread to weeds in the US (as they already have), it is only a matter of time before they spread through the rest of the world.

## Side effects of GMOs include:

1. Antibiotic resistance

There is evidence that consuming GM foods may develop antibiotic resistance in the human population. GM foods can easily change the genetic make-up of our digestive system and make us resistant to antibiotics. This would put us at risk of disease that can only be treated with antibiotics.

2. Allergies

Producers of GMOs claim that GM foods are checked for allergens and are perfectly safe to use. However, the fact that over the last 30 years, which is roughly as long as GM foods have been available in the US, there's been a dramatic increase in allergies especially in young children. This cannot be a coincidence and as soy and corn are added to many foods, especially processed foods children are so fond of, there's a very real concern that their immune systems that are still not fully developed, are being seriously compromised by GMOs.

3. Toxicity

We know that genetic modifications can trigger unexpected mutations which could make foods extremely toxic. On top of that, toxins produced by some GMOs can stay in the soil for 33 weeks (8 months) which is long enough for these toxins to join the food chain of other organisms.

Besides, in the GM plants that contain insect killer genes, the toxic material is produced continuously. It is the cumulative effect of these toxins that is a major risk to human health.

4. Cancer

Although numerous independent studies have confirmed that GMOs have carcinogenic effects, producers of GMOs claim there is not sufficient evidence these foods are a threat to human health. GM plants are resistant to pests but genetic material used to create herbicide-resistant plants (e.g., cotton, rape, soya, and corn), is known to cause cancer. GMO opponents believe that altering the plant DNA this way increases the chance of individuals using those plants as food, developing cancer.

Besides, growth hormones added to GM cattle feed, have carcinogenic effects. Needless to say, this is transferred to meat and all dairy products available in supermarkets, including baby foods.

### 5. Creation of new dangerous viruses

Viruses can get into the healthy cells and make the organism produce new copies of viruses. All genetically engineered crops contain genetic material from viruses.

The problem is that the viruses created this way could cause serious diseases for which there is no treatment.  Viruses may also cross species borders. The risk of new viruses in GM crops increases as more and more GM crops are grown.

### 6. Threats to the genetic richness

Although gene escape to the non-target organism, such as weeds or other crops, has been proven, Monsanto continues to claim that GM foods are perfectly safe. The threat that GMOs pose to biodiversity is very real since once these genes become part of the food chain, they may be impossible to get rid of and could, within years, affect the entire planet, altering and destroying biodiversity.

Still, despite all this, supporters of GMOs claim GM foods will help solve world hunger and that there is no sufficient evidence that GMOs are harmful to humans, animals, or the environment. The companies that benefit from GM food production oppose the labeling of these foods. As they have powerful lobbies, these foods are not labeled in the US and Canada.

At the same time, those who oppose GMOs claim that independent scientific research found that GM foods cause allergies, reproductive problems and infertility, organ damage, accelerated aging, insulin-regulation problems, gastrointestinal, and immune problems.

There is more than enough evidence that the rise in low-birth-weight babies, and infertility in the US population since the mid-1990s is linked to the consumption of GM foods.

GM foods include:
- 93% of soybean produced in the US, and 77% of soybean produced globally

- Close to 90% of corn produced in the US, and 26% of corn produced worldwide (this affects products such as corn syrup, canola oil, cornmeal, cornstarch, and xanthan gum).
- 95% of sugar beet grown in the US, and 9% worldwide
- 93% of cotton grown in the US, and 49% grown globally
- 80% of Hawaiian papaya is genetically modified
- 70-90% of processed foods contain GM foods
- Livestock is fed GM foods, affecting meat, milk, and eggs

Side effects as a result of GM food consumption (in humans or animals) include:

- Increased appetite and weight gain
- Changes in the immune system
- Altered intestinal structure
- Embryos with significant DNA changes
- 3rd generation lost the ability to have babies
- The high mortality of offspring
- Slower growth
- Problems with liver and kidneys
- Smaller babies
- Offspring less fertile
- Premature deliveries
- False pregnancies
- Infertility

# HOW TO IDENTIFY HYBRID AND GMO FOODS

Unless labeled as GMO, these foods usually look identical to ordinary foods. The only way to stay away from them (especially if you live in the US or Canada where GM foods are not labeled) is to know which foods are genetically modified.

GMOs can be found in:

- **Foods for human consumption**

These are soybean, corn, Innate potato, cotton, sugar beet, alfalfa, Hawaiian papaya, squash, arctic apples (these apples don't brown when cut, bruised, or bitten), and Aquabounty salmon.

## – Animal feed

These include all commercially produced meat, dairy, and eggs. Besides, cows are often injected GM growth hormones.

## – Foods that contain some GM organisms

Products made from GM foods:

a) *Canola oil and margarine*, as well as all processed foods that contain this oil. Unfortunately, this oil is added to many vegetable oils. Use olive or other healthy oils instead.

b) *GM corn* is used to make corn starch, many processed foods, and corn syrup. Sweet corn and popcorn are OK. To get around this, avoid processed foods and foods containing high fructose corn syrup.

c) *It is claimed that most GM soy* is used for animal feed and processed foods and that soy used for edamame, soy milk, tofu, and tempeh is non-GMO. This means that all processed foods that contain soy (and there are lots of them) as well as all meat, dairy, and eggs obtained from animals fed with animal feed that contains soy (all of it does) are off-limits. The only thing you can do is limit or avoid processed foods and buy only organic soy products.

d) *Most of the sugar beet* produced in the US is genetically modified, which means that when you eat processed foods that contain sugar, you are eating a GMO product. To get around this buy only organic sugar or sugar from sugar cane. Limit all food containing sugar or buy organic processed foods.

e) *US-grown papaya.*

f) Not all varieties of squash are genetically modified, so check which ones are from the Monsanto seed catalog or buy organic squash.

g) Salmon is the first animal to be genetically modified. All processed foods containing salmon are usually made from GM salmon. Avoid eating salmon as well as all processed foods containing salmon.

# LIST OF PLANT-BASED HYBRID FOODS

Hundreds of plants have been hybridized over the last couple of hundred years, however, in the case of some of those plants, there is no scientific evidence which plants were used to create certain hybrids.

Some of the most common hybridized plants that we know which plants they were hybridized from include:

- Kiwi
- Sisal
- Great headed garlic
- Pineapple
- Peanut
- Oat
- Hemp
- Pecan
- Chestnut
- Radicchio
- Key lime
- Lemon
- Sour oranges
- Clementine
- Grapefruit
- Mandarin
- Sweet orange
- Coconut
- Coffee
- Hazelnut
- Carrot
- Yam
- Strawberry
- Barley
- Hops
- Walnut
- Macadamia
- Apple
- Peppermint
- Banana
- Tobacco
- Avocado
- Pea
- Cherry

- Plum
- Almond
- Pear
- Radish
- Raspberry
- Sugar cane
- Rye
- Millet
- Potato
- Tomato (Except Plum and Cherry)
- Eggplant
- Cacao
- Spelt
- Durum wheat
- Vanilla
- Grapes
- Maize (corn)

# CHAPTER 3: ABOUT DR. SEBI – THE MAN, HIS LIFE AND TEACHINGS

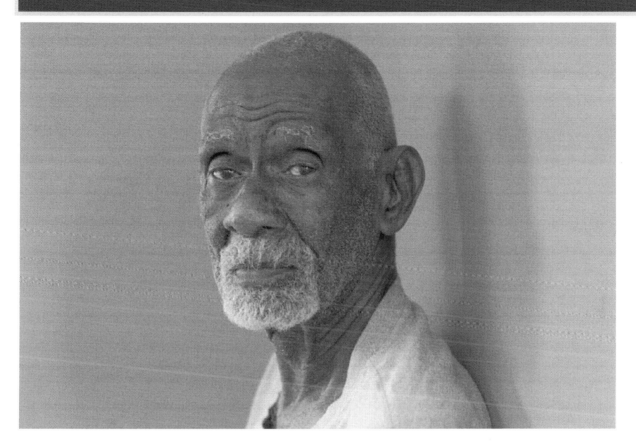

Dr. Sebi (real names: Alfredo Darington Bowman) was a Honduran herbalist, naturalist and healer. Although, he didn't have formal medical training, he helped a lot of people cure the most serious health conditions. His secret was an alkaline electric based diet and herbal remedies. Born in 1933, Dr. Sebi learned from his grandmother, "Mama Hay," and subsequently, in curing himself of diabetes, asthma, and impotency with a herbalist in Mexico. After getting healed through herbs, Dr Sebi created his unique line of natural cell food compounds that he used for cleansing and revitalization.

Dr. Sebi's approach to disease relies on the theory of the African bio-mineral balance and herbal remedies to cleanse and detoxify the body, returning it to its previous intended alkaline state – a state which is free from disease.

## HISTORY

Dr. Sebi developed his healing methodology after an herbalist in Mexico helped him cure him of asthma, diabetes, and impotence. Although he had some basic knowledge of herbalism, it was after the visit to the Mexican herbalist that made him realize that even the most serious health conditions could be avoided or treated with a change of diet and herbal remedies. He has helped quite a lot of people who were written off by conventional medicine.

Dr. Sebi spent decades studying the plants and herbs of North, South and Central America, Africa and the Caribbean. Born in 1933, Dr. Sebi learned from his grandmother, "Mama Hay," and subsequently, in curing himself of diabetes, asthma, and impotency with a herbalist in Mexico. After getting healed through herbs, Dr Sebi created his unique line of natural cell food compounds that he used for cleansing and revitalization. Dr. Sebi's approach to disease relies on the theory of the African bio-mineral balance. He relies on herbal remedies to cleanse and detoxify the body, returning it to its previous intended alkaline state – a state which is free from disease.

When his healing method became well known world-wide, Dr. Sebi opened up healing practices first in Honduras, followed by New York and Los Angeles. However, because he did not have a license to practice as a healer, New York charged him with a criminal charge of working without a license. He was acquitted but was soon sued again for claiming he had a cure for AIDS, cancer, leukemia, lupus, and other untreatable diseases. In 2016 Dr. Sebi was arrested in Honduras but after falling sick while in prison and not receiving adequate treatment, he died of pneumonia-related complications. Dr. Sebi's methodology is based on an alkaline diet and healing methodology which he termed "The African Bio-Mineral Balance". His remedies are mainly based on herbs from North America, Central and South America, Africa, and the Caribbean.

## ABOUT THE NAME – DR. SEBI

Dr Sebi was a self-educated herbalist and naturalist who healed many with chronic conditions. Many of these patients have proclaimed their unbelievable healing experience with Dr. Sebi's healing methodology. His wife Maa gave him the name Sebi and locals began calling him Doctor Sebi after they saw him heal fatal illnesses.

## DR. SEBI ON HIS HEALING IN MEXICO

Dr. Sebi developed his healing methodology after the Mexican herbalist helped him cure him of asthma, diabetes, and impotence. After he was healed, the herbalist advised Dr. Sebi to avoid foods such as meat, lamb and milk. It cured him and he lived for more than 82 years.

*Hear Dr. Sebi Speak:*

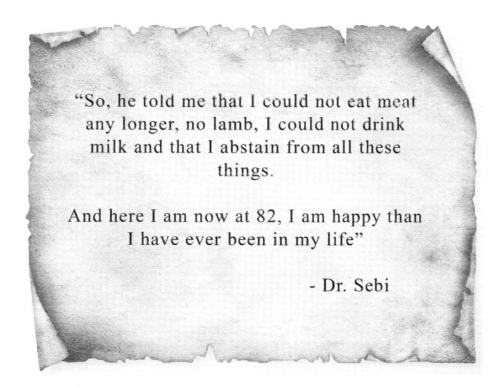

"So, he told me that I could not eat meat any longer, no lamb, I could not drink milk and that I abstain from all these things.

And here I am now at 82, I am happy than I have ever been in my life"

- Dr. Sebi

## DR. SEBI ON HIS FIRST CURE

Dr. Sebi spent decades studying the plants and herbs of North, South and Central America, Africa and the Caribbean. After the successful treatment from the herbalist, Dr. Sebi researched on herbs all over the world and finally he found plants which could treat diseases like Herpes, AIDS, and many other diseases termed "incurable." At the very beginning, he treated his own brother Michael White who lived in Boston. Dr. Sebi recommended him a diet free from lactose, uric acid, carbonic acid – which were milk, meat and starches in that order.

***Hear Dr. Sebi Speak:***

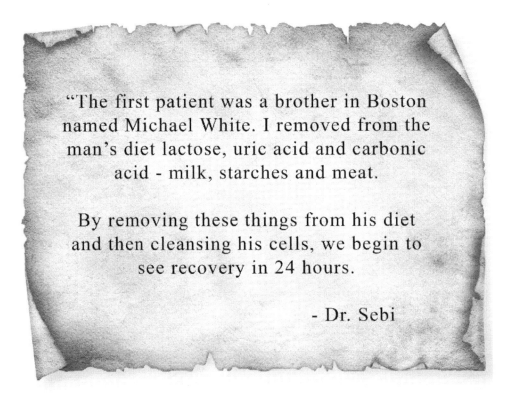

"The first patient was a brother in Boston named Michael White. I removed from the man's diet lactose, uric acid and carbonic acid - milk, starches and meat.

By removing these things from his diet and then cleansing his cells, we begin to see recovery in 24 hours.

- Dr. Sebi

After removing these "substances" from his diet, he was able to cleanse his cells and he began to see recovery. He subsequently cured many others including around 13 patients who suffered with AIDS.

## DR. SEBI ON THE FEDERAL ALLEGATIONS

When his healing method became well known world-wide, Dr. Sebi opened up healing practices first in Honduras, followed by New York and Los Angeles. Dr. Sebi treated Herpes, cancer, AIDS, sickle-cell, lupus, blindness and many other diseases. So, in early 1980, the food and drug administration charged him with practicing medication without a license. He had chance to prove himself to judges and perform a trial where treated patients who suffered from each disease. He was acquitted but was soon sued again for claiming he had a cure for AIDS, cancer, leukemia, lupus, and other untreatable diseases.

But did he defend himself?

**_Hear Dr. Sebi explain:_**

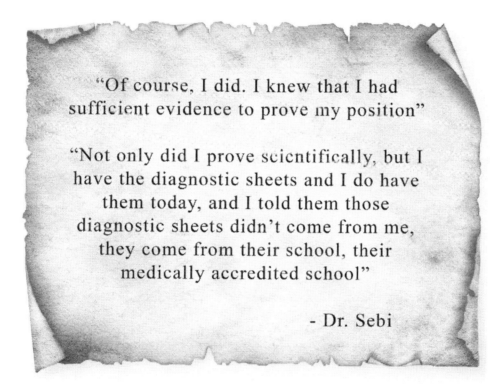

"Of course, I did. I knew that I had sufficient evidence to prove my position"

"Not only did I prove scientifically, but I have the diagnostic sheets and I do have them today, and I told them those diagnostic sheets didn't come from me, they come from their school, their medically accredited school"

- Dr. Sebi

Those patients had to bring reports before the treatment from a doctor and after the treatment from a separate doctor. Finally, Dr. Sebi accomplished the trials and proved that he could cure the incurable diseases. He did this by treating 70 patients. In fact, there was no need to attend the court proceedings because the patients came along with verified medical reports which showed that they had been cured by Dr. Sebi's treatments.

Dr. Sebi was interviewed by doctors and they decided there was no fault because all his treatments were based on essential foods. So, Dr. Sebi was found not guilty after presenting himself to the Attorney General. Also, Dr. Sebi's medicines, cell compounds and products were made from fig tree and it had been proven as electric cell-food by the Lancaster Laboratories who conducted research on those compounds on the court's order. After the legal victory, Dr. Sebi became a famous healer in the community and many of his patients cured with his medicine gave testimonies.

Although he had some basic knowledge of herbalism, it was after his visit to the Mexican herbalist that made him realize that even the most serious health conditions could be avoided or treated with a change of diet and herbal remedies. He has helped quite a lot of people who were written off by conventional medicine.

## DR. SEBI ON HIS HEALING METHODOLOGY

*How did Dr. Sebi say he was healing people of these incurable diseases?*

Dr. Sebi's treatments were based on removing excess mucus from the body and he believed that the mucus is the cause of every disease. He explained that deposition of these toxic mucus beyond the limits causes disease or inflammation. For example, excess mucus in the bronchial tube causes Bronchitis and excess mucus in the joints causes Arthritis.

**Hear Dr. Sebi:**

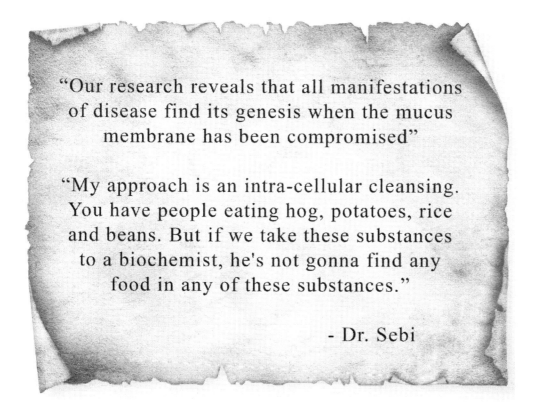

"Our research reveals that all manifestations of disease find its genesis when the mucus membrane has been compromised"

"My approach is an intra-cellular cleansing. You have people eating hog, potatoes, rice and beans. But if we take these substances to a biochemist, he's not gonna find any food in any of these substances."

- Dr. Sebi

Dr. Sebi's theory was based on an alkaline diet. He posited that an alkaline diet does not cause formation of excess mucus. Instead, it cleanses the body and that it is electrical and contains the most beneficial materials for human body. These substances that are electrical can be found in nature. This is so because their molecular structure has not been tampered with.

So, Dr. Sebi believed that, once a person becomes a vegetarian, all the diseases which caused pain will be healed.

**He explains:**

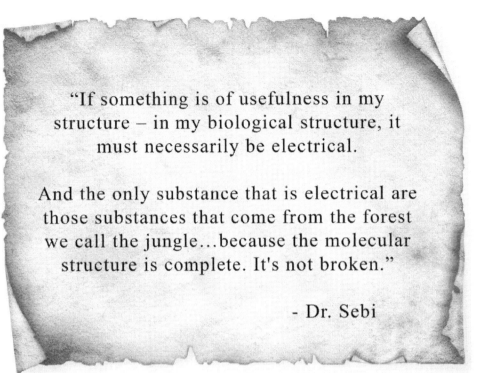

"If something is of usefulness in my structure – in my biological structure, it must necessarily be electrical.

And the only substance that is electrical are those substances that come from the forest we call the jungle...because the molecular structure is complete. It's not broken."

- Dr. Sebi

Dr. Sebi explains that electric foods are medicine in itself and they help the human body to heal, rebuild and nourish itself. They are alkaline and found in nature. They are not hybrid, irradiated, or genetically-modified. Electric foods improve the electrical activity in the nerves and helps with better cognitive function. It boosts your mental clarity and use of one's senses. Electricity is the reason the human body can move - crawl, walk, climb or run. Without electricity, there would be no movement and no life. If the body is electric, then you should feed it electric (alkaline) nutrition. Electric foods are made in nature, non-hybridized and non-GMO. They are mostly found wild in nature – in the jungle and grown without the use of chemical fertilizers and pesticides.

## DR. SEBI ON BLACK HEALTH

The overall consensus is that there's but ONE race - the human race.  That basically, we're the same.  Race is regarded as a social concept used to create difference and the illusion of inequality.  However, the reality is, we're not the same.  There's a physiological and biological difference in all races.  And that distinction is what we call MELANIN.  As a black person, you're distinct. You are different.  You're unique, special, and strong unlike any other racial group.  It's very important that Black women understand the fundamentals about melanin and the best way to nourish it.  This is sacrosanct and very important to sustain the physical, spiritual and mental wellbeing of our existence. We must understand this so we can better the health we so desperately need in our own lives and communities.

So, what's Melanin?  Dr. Llaila Afrika clarifies that Melanin is the "*biochemical component that compels physical, psychological, psychological and religious life*".  Melanin is a natural dark carbon compound substance that is found available in every tissue, cell, and organ within the body.  It is not only present in our skin or eyes, it's in our nerves, reproductive, digestive and circulatory systems.  Melanin modulates all physiological functions, cycles, circadian rhythms, and glands in the human body.  Melanin is the driving force of our sleep and wake cycle. Melanin is life. All races have melanin; however, black individuals have the largest concentration of melanin.  Melanin is readily visible in our skin, eyes, skin, and hair. Melanin is also, as Dr. Afrika says "*What makes black people black*". Melanin is the reason we could create ancient civilizations, build the pyramids, establish booming cultures, produce greats in the areas of astrology, medicine, mathematics, and technology. Melanin is why we survived the chattel slavery and Middle Passage. Melanin is the reason this nation was built; together with all the blood, tears, sweat and strength of our ancestors.  Melanin is why Ossie Davis states, "*I find, in being black, something of beauty: a pleasure; a power; a key cup of gladness.*" Melanin is our ability, our intellect, our creativity, and our power.

This is why we must nourish melanin- not just for self-preservation, but for health, peace, harmony and the love of nature. When Black people nourish their melanin correctly, they can heal themselves in half the time as melanin-diminished people.  When black people nourish their melanin properly, they're more resilient, versatile, effective, have more mental clarity, enhanced cognitive functioning, improved health, and a general improved outlook in life.

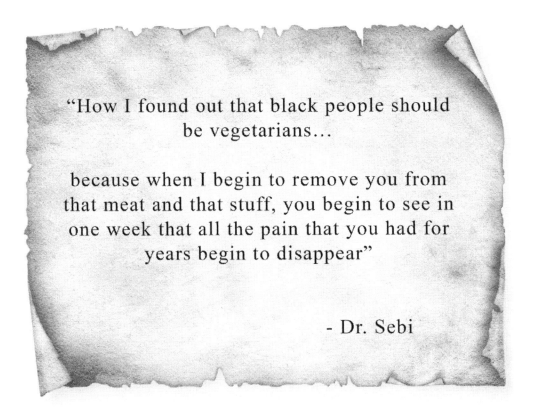

"How I found out that black people should be vegetarians...

because when I begin to remove you from that meat and that stuff, you begin to see in one week that all the pain that you had for years begin to disappear"

- Dr. Sebi

As Black people, we have to understand this very important fundamental. We have to know that we're not similar. We can't eat, think, or live our lives in a way that dishonors who we are. We're a melanin dominant race and we must live our lives with all the knowledge and understanding of the role melanin plays in our own lives. We have to sever ties with the Standard American Diet, Western contemporary medication, and Eurocentric methods of living and thinking that reduce or diminishes the ability of melanin in our own lives.

## DR. SEBI ON THE GERM THEORY OF DISEASE

Dr. Sebi did not believe on germs such as viruses or bacteria - which was contrary to basic science. Dr. Sebi ignored all criticisms and continued his career. He said that western medicine had become a norm which unfortunately could not allow people to think about other possible ways.

**Hear Dr. Sebi Speak:**

"At the Supreme Court in the United States, the judge said: What did you say?

I said there is no such thing as a germ, a virus or a bacterium.

Then what is it?
I said it is a microbe that is generated in the body when *erosion* begins."

- Dr. Sebi

"If I take a very healthy human being and lay them on this table and not move them for a month, when
I raise them what are they gonna have on the back?
...there would be some little worms, but where did the worms come from and where were they born?
Inside that man who is healthy. Why is that so? That part of the body was lacking of oxygen"

- Dr. Sebi

Before thinking about healing, we must first understand the cause of disease. Why do we get sick.? *Or better put*, why do we get *so* sick *today*? We are now conditioned to believe that dirt is harmful and that most diseases come from germs present in the soil and dirt. But you think about this critically, you'll see that our forebears lived with the soil and lived long. Our forefathers and ancestors didn't live in polished or titled living rooms. Their feet and bodies were in constant contact with dirt and soil. And they didn't get sick! They lived long until old age.

Dr. Sebi himself told us he came from an organic family. A family that lives on natural foods and herbs. As a little boy he'd say, their sewer system was right beside their living room. And they never got sick. They would poop and use it as manure. They didn't get scared of illness.

Like Dr. Sebi said, we get sick because our mucus membranes become compromised. Now, the next question should be, what compromises this structure? What's violates this biological structure? It's just common sense to deduct that if our forebears lived so long on dirt and soil, dirt shouldn't be the cause of disease. Ever since I discovered that dirt is never the problem, I roll in soil, at the beach and the garden. I walk barefoot! You'll never can imagine that feeling of skin on soil. And guess what? I sleep like a log afterwards. We must think and understand this. Disease is way beyond viruses and bacteria and fungi.

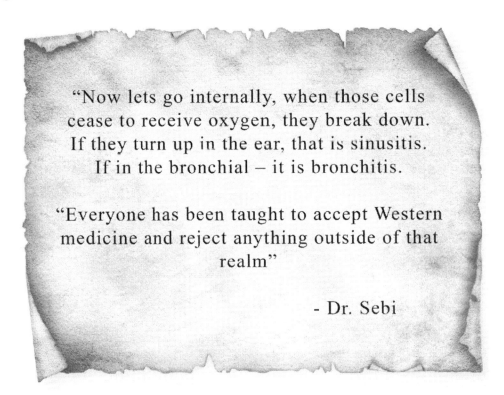

"Now lets go internally, when those cells cease to receive oxygen, they break down. If they turn up in the ear, that is sinusitis. If in the bronchial – it is bronchitis.

"Everyone has been taught to accept Western medicine and reject anything outside of that realm"

- Dr. Sebi

We have shielded ourselves so much away from dirt and soil. We do so because we believe viruses and bacteria and fungi present their cause disease. Conventional medicine tells us so. But what if they're wrong. Is dirt really that bad? Could it be worse that the chemical antibiotics they give us? Could dirt be worse than the alcohol, sugar, synthetic salt and all other poisonous foods we invest into our system in the name of food.

Disease is more to do with a compromised body system, a compromised immunity! We can take HIV or Herpes for example. HIV do not cause you disease. It only weakens your system. It is your weakened immune system that gives way for disease to invade you. But HIV will do no harm if you stay true to natural alkaline medicine. Yes. That's because the protection and barrier true herbal medicine gives is more than any attacking force from any viral agents.

## DR. SEBI ON HOLISTIC HEALING

Dr Sebi's talent in healing patients with chronic diseases, led people to trust him and proclaim him as a doctor. Dr. Sebi experimented on himself by consuming rare herbs and also fasting for long time. Not only did he use herbs, he also used several other techniques to heal. Those spiritual and psychological treatments were based on changing the way of thinking, improving self-confidence and independent living.

## DR. SEBI ON HEALING BLINDNESS

Dr. Sebi treated a blind patient with his compounds and his nutritional guide. Later he explained, that the patient told him he had been trying to heal for 11 years but he failed and that if Sebi could cure him, it would be a miracle. So, after several days, the patient gained his sight with the help of Dr. Sebi's medicine made out of alkaline herbs.

*Hear Dr. Sebi:*

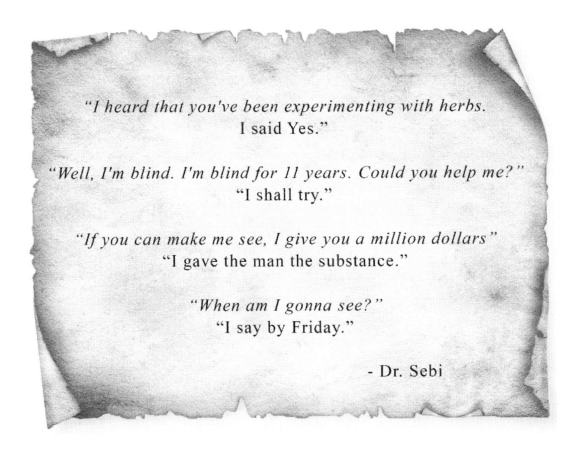

*"I heard that you've been experimenting with herbs. I said Yes."*

*"Well, I'm blind. I'm blind for 11 years. Could you help me?"*
"I shall try."

*"If you can make me see, I give you a million dollars"*
"I gave the man the substance."

*"When am I gonna see?"*
"I say by Friday."

- Dr. Sebi

Many would think blindness just like AIDS and Herpes is incurable. But that isn't. There are enough evidences that show that there is no incurable diseases. Everything the human race needs for health and healing is found in nature.

We have sinned against nature and that's why we have disease. We have you go back to the roots to seek and understand true healing to disease. We have to preserve our genome. The African Biomineral balance theory teaches us this. That's the only way to stop or prevent disease. We must understand the true reason we get sick before we can know how to cure to heal from it. Once we know this, it's the first step towards healing. There is no way a diabetic who is seeking to heal and do not know that he needs to stop eating the way he did in time past. He would first learn by retrospect why he got the disease and then practice

"Now why did I select Friday until this day?
I don't know. But I was so sure of myself.
How did a boy who didn't go to school be so sure of himself. The man went home with the medicine."

"And on Wednesday, Good morning young man.
I raised my right hand and he said *you raised your right hand*. I winked my left eye, and he said *you winked your left eye*."

"I said the man is seeing. At that point of my journey, I could explain that I know it's a bunch of herbs that cleansed the man's body but they were all alkaline plants."

- Dr. Sebi

## DR. SEBI'S METHOD OF CLEANSE AND REVITALIZING

Dr. Sebi's method of cleanse and revitalizing can be used by anyone with a disease or whoever needs to revitalize the body. There are several processes that should be undertaken during this process. Cleansing the body by consuming spring water, herbs, alkaline fruit smoothies, tamarind, Irish moss, and green juice. And then fasting followed by consuming herbs that boost the immune system.

When these steps are followed, the body starts to heal. This healing typically happens in two steps – the first step is intra-cellular detoxification and elimination of mucus. This is generally referred to as "Cleansing of the body." The second step is restoring the body's lost energy and balance by consuming sea moss and revitalizing herbs.

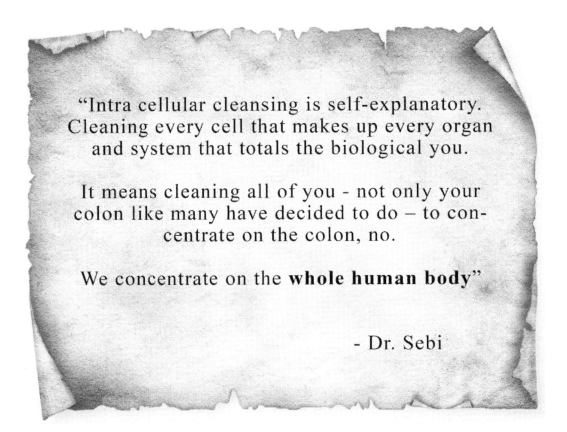

"Intra cellular cleansing is self-explanatory. Cleaning every cell that makes up every organ and system that totals the biological you.

It means cleaning all of you - not only your colon like many have decided to do – to concentrate on the colon, no.

We concentrate on the **whole human body**"

- Dr. Sebi

Dr Sebi mentioned that cleansing should be holistic and cover all parts of the body including the organs like skin, liver, gall bladder, lymph glands, kidney, and colon. Unfortunately, many people only concentrate on the colon.

After the cleanse, revitalization is next. It is basically a process of restoring the energy that was lost due to the disease. Basically, energy is replaced with minerals like phosphates and iron which are electrical in nature. To get electrical minerals, Dr. Sebi advised to consume electrical herbs which are the base ingredients of his products.

> "Cleansing the human body is only about one part of the whole journey; the other is bringing back the energy that was lost by the presence of disease.
>
> That energy is supported by minerals – live minerals - phosphates of iron, phosphate of calcium and phosphates of everything that we're going to use will have to be phosphate.
>
> Why? Because they and they alone are electrical."
>
> - Dr. Sebi

Detoxification is removing toxins which accumulated in the body. The common method of detoxification is fasting and there are several types of fasting methods such as raw food fast, smoothie fasting, water fasting, liquid fasting and fruit fasting.

Dr. Sebi recommended to fast for at least 12 days with sea moss, herbs, water, or fruit or veggie smoothies. This method of fasting entails consuming the selected food or liquid along with the detoxing herbs. During the detoxification process, there may be different signs and symptoms you may notice like mucus, lower blood pressure, pains, itching, flu and cold, difficulty in sleeping, etc. Those signs however disappear after first week of detoxification.

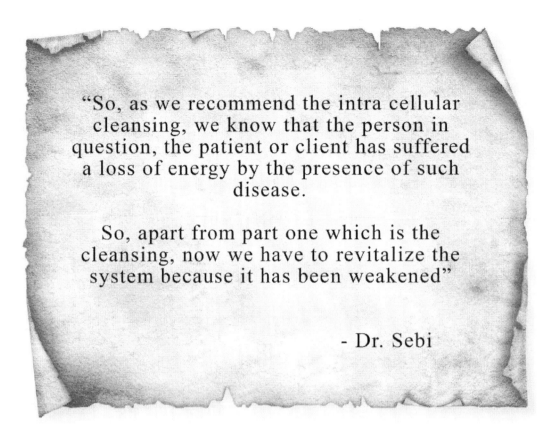

"So, as we recommend the intra cellular cleansing, we know that the person in question, the patient or client has suffered a loss of energy by the presence of such disease.

So, apart from part one which is the cleansing, now we have to revitalize the system because it has been weakened"

- Dr. Sebi

The detoxification process may vary from person to person and on toxic level in the body. Normally it is recommended to use one to two weeks, but one to three months of fasting will give good results. Minimum time period for fasting is 12 days. If the person is suffering from any disease, the detoxification process may take more time than a normal healthier person. Anyone with any disease that cannot fast on water or juice, should follow fruit or raw vegetable fasting according to the Dr. Sebi's nutritional guide.

## DR. SEBI ON ELECTRIC ALKALINE HERBS

Dr. Sebi studied herbs from Africa, North and South America, and Europe and focused his research and healing methodology on acid/alkaline balance within a human body. However, he did not base his therapies only on alkaline foods. He went a step further. He was adamant that all hybridized herbs (and foods) should be excluded from a healthy diet.

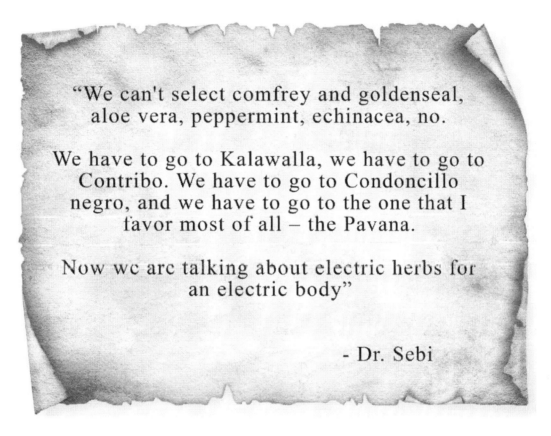

"We can't select comfrey and goldenseal, aloe vera, peppermint, echinacea, no.

We have to go to Kalawalla, we have to go to Contribo. We have to go to Condoncillo negro, and we have to go to the one that I favor most of all – the Pavana.

Now we are talking about electric herbs for an electric body"

- Dr. Sebi

Dr. Sebi insisted that alkaline herbs are essential for health and vitality and was very passionate about which herbs support one's health and which ones don't. His approach to herbalism was based on a belief that only that which is natural, can be truly healing. Most of the foods available today (ie fruits, vegetables, herbs, spices, grains, etc) were at some stage cross-bred to improve the yield. The list of all hybridized plants is too long to mention but the problem with this is that some of the herbs not approved by Dr. Sebi are unfortunately touted in the health community to have amazing health benefits, e.g. Aloe Vera, Echinacea, ginseng, turmeric, mint, ginger, garlic, etc. Dr. Sebi insisted they are hybrid and acidic and should be excluded from diet.

Dr. Sebi based his approach on the simple premise that wild plants were created in God's laboratory, while hybridized plants were created in medical laboratories through cross-pollination and genetic modification. As a result, they have an incomplete molecular structure. They are acid-based and should not be consumed for the simple reason that they are unnatural. According to Dr. Sebi, hybridized herbs and foods are acid-forming and negatively affect the brain (eg mint), destroy cells by weakening their membranes (eg garlic). If you are trying to heal using Dr. Sebi methodology, you should stay away from them.

## THE USHA INSTITUTE

After the court occurrence in the 1980's, Dr. Sebi built a village called USHA which he named after his oldest daughter. That healing place is situated in Honduras in Central America and many people visited to have treatments for different diseases. At the beginning, Dr. Sebi spent his time in Usha village with his family but now it is managed by his former business partners.

## DR. SEBI ON CELEBRITIES – LISA "LEFT-EYE" LOPEZ, MICHAEL JACKSON, STEVEN SEAGAL AND NIPSEY HUSSLE

Several famous celebrities were treated by Dr. Sebi including Lisa Lopes, John Travolta, Eddie Murphy, Michael Jackson and Nipsey Hussle. Lisa Lopez is a famous character who got cured with Dr. Sebi's treatments. He had mentioned this in one of his interviews. She spent time in Usha village and went through several medications - those medications by Dr. Sebi cured her which she had struggled with in her day-to-day life.

**Dr. Sebi says:**

"She told me she was suffering with alcoholism and she was smoking excessive cigarettes - Drinking and smoking. She asked me: *what do I need to do to stay on the side of Peace?*

I said fast. Do what Jesus did.
And she said what did Jesus do? He fasted for 40 days and 40 nights.

At at the end of the fasting, she came to me, I heard the door opening at 2 o'clock in the morning, she said I completed my fast this morning.
I asked what did you see?
*I saw God* she said"

\- Dr. Sebi

Lisa Lopes was highly addicted to alcohol and smoking and she asked for help from Dr. Sebi. Dr. Sebi advised her to go on a fast for 40 days and she did. At the end of the fast, she felt really healthy as she stated "I saw the god".

Lisa Lopez talked about her experience and she shared it with her fans through the media. She wanted people in same predicament as she was to get relief. Lisa Lopes died in a car accident and rumors had it that she was killed.

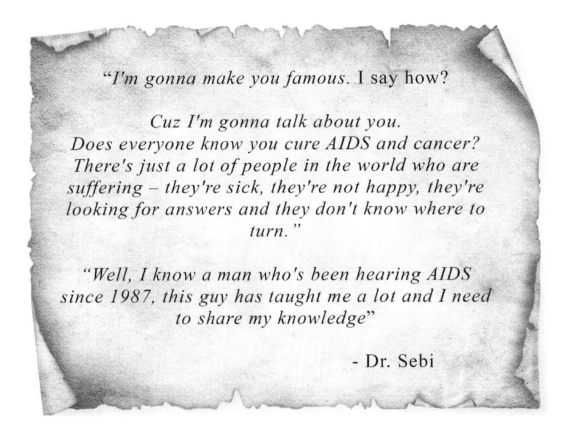

"*I'm gonna make you famous. I say how?*

*Cuz I'm gonna talk about you.*
*Does everyone know you cure AIDS and cancer?*
*There's just a lot of people in the world who are*
*suffering – they're sick, they're not happy, they're*
*looking for answers and they don't know where to*
*turn.*"

"*Well, I know a man who's been hearing AIDS*
*since 1987, this guy has taught me a lot and I need*
*to share my knowledge*"

- Dr. Sebi

Several other celebrities were also treated by Dr. Sebi. Nipsey Hussle made a statement that he was going to make a documentary on Dr. Sebi's healing methodology but in 2019 he was murdered. There are rumors that Nipsey Hussle was murdered because he of his above statement which scared some people that Dr. Sebi's cure could become famous.

Dr. Sebi treated Michael Jackson who was heavily addicted to drugs. Those drugs damaged his nerves and Dr. Sebi did intra-cellular chelation which healed him. In the case of Steven Seagal, Dr. Sebi cured his long-time headache with his treatments. There are people who condemned Dr. Sebi as a scam because of his several theories on glucose and germs. According to Dr. Sebi, glucose can cause excess fat and not good for human health. But some people who were against Dr. Sebi, pointed out that the glucose is the basic energy source of human.

## DR. SEBI FAMILY LIFE

Dr Sebi was a passionate person who had four marriages, although three of them were presumed not legal. His first wife was Melba Jean followed by Maa,

Annette Thomas, and finally Pasty. Dr. Sebi started his first outlet in the Caribbean Island with Maa and where he met Annette Thomas later.

Dr. Sebi opened his next outlet in New York. After many years Pasty moved to ocean village and started to serve Dr. Sebi. Maa separated from Dr. Sebi because of his other relationships and she continue her treatments with her children. Dr. Sebi later moved to Los Angles and married Pasty who helped him further.  Together they opened a new company there. These 4 marriages produced more than 20 children.

## DR. SEBI'S DEATH

Dr. Sebi was arrested because of money laundering and his family tried hard to get him released but they were not successful. He was kept in jail for months and suffered with pneumonia during this period. Some of his family members had alleged that Dr. Sebi was starved in jail and murdered. His postmortem report was not released.  Dr. Sebi's daughter Usha said that there were several evidences, but investigation on her father's murder case was not released.

She also explained that at the last telephonic conversation with her father, he had mention that someone trying to kill him. Dr. Sebi's family members understood that he was a threat to western medicine and pharmaceutical industries and it didn't come as surprise if they tried to silence him.

## DR. SEBI, POST-DEATH

An incident occurred where a young man had allergy on his head. After applying one of Dr. Sebi's products, he had posted the controversial results on social media. This caused rejection of Dr. Sebi's product by some people. But Dr. Sebi's family members warned there were lots of fake products and fake social media accounts which often used Dr. Sebi's identity. One of Dr. Sebi's assistant sold such products using Dr. Sebi's identity.

Also, there were several conflicts among the family members on Dr. Sebi's properties and products. Pasty Bowman, Dr. Sebi's legal wife owns the international healing and Dr. Sebi's authentic product and she mentioned that she and Dr. Sebi's second wife Maa had the original products. But many of Dr. Sebi's customers believe that the original products can be purchased from Greenleaf herbal solutions owned by Dr. Sebi's third wife Annette Thomas and that those were the products which he used in his very first trail at the court. In several other interviews, Dr. Sebi's had mentioned that His wife, ex-wives, and his children betrayed him.

# CHAPTER 4: THE DR. SEBI ALKALINE DIET HEALING METHODOLOGY

## GOALS OF DR. SEBI HEALING METHODOLOGY

### 1. To Cleanse/Detox

According to Dr. Sebi;

*"Disease can only exist in an environment that is acid...only consistent use of natural botanical remedies will effectively cleanse and detoxify diseased body, reversing it to its intended alkaline state.*

Dr. Sebi insisted on using only natural electric herbs to heal the body. These herbs cleanse the cells on the cellular and intra-cellular level. Only natural herbs can replenish our bodies and keep in tune with our electric bodies. The food we eat today is unfortunately based on acidic foods, e.g. meat, dairy, sugar, etc. Today's diet is typically western, it is so high in processed, GMO, and hybridized foods which unbalance the alkalinity of the blood. Dr. Sebi advised to avoid all these foods and eat only natural foods made my God.

Dr. Sebi healing method revolves around the idea that disease exists only in an acidic environment. Therefore, his motto was: alkalize the environment and get rid of the disease. We know that the body constantly tries to maintain a healthy balance of 7.4 pH level in the blood. We can help it achieve and maintain this balance if we eat a natural alkaline based electric diet. Unfortunately, a typical western diet is high in very acidic foods. It is tasty, convenient, and nutrient deficient.

### 2. To revitalize the body

Dr. Sebi protocol is based on the idea that the reason the western diet is unhealthy is that, being heavily processed, it lacks nutrition. That's why he insisted on foods that include over 100 minerals that support electrical activity and overall vitality of the body.

# PRINCIPLES OF DR. SEBI ALKALINE DIET

Dr. Sebi diet is based on the following principles:

## 1.  1. You must only eat foods listed on the Dr. Sebi Food list

Eat only the foods that are on the Dr. Sebi food list. The list is very specific (and restrictive) and excludes many nutritious foods. Dr. Sebi believed strongly in natural foods and insisted one should stay away from hybridized fruits and vegetables (i.e., plants produced by unnatural cross-pollination). He was adamant that these foods have their genetic structure, electrical composition, and pH balance changed and are therefore not suitable for human consumption.

Dr. Sebi insisted that you eat only the foods from his list of approved foods. Although the list is quite restrictive and many foods are left out, it contains wholly natural alkaline foods. Besides, Dr. Sebi insisted that no hybridized foods should be taken. By hybridized foods, he meant all the plants produced by artificial cross-pollination. Needless to say, most of the fruits and vegetables available today are hybridized. Although Dr. Sebi diet seems rather restrictive, you can still create healthy, balanced, and tasty meals with the approved foods. One of the reasons so many foods have been left out from the list is that so much of what we eat today is hybridized. Dr. Sebi believed that although hybridized fruits and vegetables generally taste better than the original plants they were developed from, their nutrient level is lower. One of the ways to know a plant that is hybridized is if it has no seeds. We now have quite a lot of seedless fruits ranging from watermelon, oranges, grapes, to tomatoes and berries. etc. Avoid these whenever you can. Dr. Sebi believed that natural foods are much healthier than those created by man.

## 2.  Drink Springwater

According to Dr. Sebi method, you should drink about 4 liters (1 gallon) of natural spring water a day because it helps flush out accumulated toxins. Many of the herbs from Dr. Sebi Food list are diuretics that increase urination. Toxins are naturally flushed out through urine, stool, and sweat.

Drinking about 4 liters of water a day is necessary partly because 70% of our body is water, and partly because water helps with the detoxification process.

Waste that remains in the body for too long (eg when you are constipated) becomes toxic. Water also helps with the absorption of nutrients. This is why many of the herbs Dr. Sebi recommends are diuretics that increase urination and so help remove toxins from the body. Springwater may not be easy to come by nowadays but it provides the best hydration.

## 3. No microwaving

Dr. Sebi considered food prepared in microwave unhealthy and recommended the use of a stove or oven for heating or cooking your meals. An ideal solution would be eating raw foods whenever possible.

Dr. Sebi was convinced that microwaving is a very unhealthy method of food preparation and insisted one used a stove for cooking.

## 4. No Canned and Seedless fruits

Many of the seedless fruits available today are hybridized. There is hardly a naturally occurring seedless fruit. Canned foods also contain a lot of added sugar and preservatives such as salt. The reason for this is understandable.

## 5. No Animal Products (Meat, Fish, Eggs, Dairy, Honey, GMO's)

## 6. No Sugar (White and brown)

## 7. No Alcohol

Dr. Sebi believed that with the alkaline diet it's possible to both prevent and cure disease. According to him, the disease is a result of mucus build-up in an area of your body. For example, a build-up of mucus in the lungs causes pneumonia, while excess mucus in the pancreas leads to diabetes, etc.

Dr. Sebi argued that diseases cannot exist in an alkaline environment and only occur when your body becomes too acidic. He believed that by strictly following his diet and using the prescribed supplements, it's possible to restore your body's ideal pH levels and get rid of the accumulated toxins.

Dr. Sebi alkaline diet comprises of a list of approved fruits, vegetables, grains, seeds, herbs, nuts and oils. He claimed that for your body to heal itself, and stay healthy, you must follow the diet consistently for the rest of your life.

# DR. SEBI ELECTRIC DIET VS CONVENTIONAL DIET

The concept of the alkaline diet is not a new one. It's been known since the middle of the 19-th century. Although some of the aspects of the alkaline diet were used by many nutritionists and holistic practitioners, the alkaline diet became popular relatively recently. It was during the 1990s, that some nutritionists started suggesting a 100% alkaline diet. Dr. Sebi took this a step further. He developed a diet that revolved around maintaining vitality by using the "African Bio Mineral Balance". Dr. Sebi referred to his method as either the African Bio-mineral balance or the African Bio Balance. The African Bio-mineral Balance remedy consists of 102 minerals that support electrical activity and overall vitality of the body. This therapeutic approach addresses disease on two levels. It first cleanses the body of acidity. This step relies heavily on herbs that clean the body's cells on both the cellular and intra-cellular level. The next step is to revitalize cells by supplying minerals that have been lost through the consumption of acidic foods.

Unfortunately, 90% of the modern diet is based on acidic foods, e.g. meat, dairy, processed foods as well as GMO and hybridized foods. Eating these foods will acidify the body and unbalance the alkalinity of the blood. The reason Dr. Sebi insisted on unhybridized fruits and vegetables is that such foods have an alkaline base. They were designed by nature to provide a human body with all it needs for optimal health. Dr. Sebi developed his approach to health on the assumption that disease can only exist in an acidic environment. The body works non-stop to maintain a 7.4 pH level in the blood. When you eat a balanced diet, your body is perfectly capable of maintaining this level of acidity. However, the modern diet is very unbalanced. It is based on carbs, meat, sugar, and junk food which are all very acidic and which is why our body needs help to maintain homeostasis.

Some of the cleansing herbs Dr. Sebi used in his alkaline diet are burdock root, sarsaparilla, and dandelion, which clean the blood and the liver. Dr. Sebi diet revolves around three principles that are simple to follow and that everyone can easily fit into their lifestyle, no matter how hectic or unusual.

# CHAPTER 5: HOW TO GET STARTED ON THE DR. SEBI DIET AS A BEGINNER

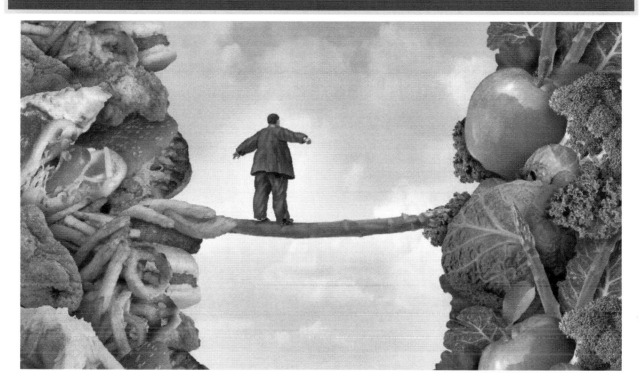

Alkaline foods are some of the healthiest foods there are, and they are particularly recommended to those suffering from frequent colds, headaches, low energy, anxiety, and benign breast and ovarian cysts. The foods that are known to contribute to acid and that we usually eat a lot of are red meat, pasta, sweets, and dairy. Changing a diet, especially if it is supposed to be a drastic change, is not easy. To improve your health, you have to find a way of reducing the acid load and adopting healthier eating habits.

## HOW TO GRADUALLY SWITCH TO THE DR. SEBI ALKALINE-ANTI-INFLAMMATORY DIET

Many people don't enjoy dieting but the best results are achieved when the desire to change your eating habits is self-imposed, rather than suggested by someone else, e.g., doctor, colleague, partner, etc. It's best to proceed slowly and set a goal, e.g., to lower your cholesterol levels. However, what seems to be even more difficult from changing a diet is maintaining it. Most diets are to a certain degree restrictive and although most people usually stick to a diet for a while, i.e., until they've achieved their goals, e.g., to lose a certain amount of weight, what everyone finds very difficult is sticking to a new dietary regimen for extended periods.

One of the methods for a "smooth transition" is that, before going on a diet, you start eating healthy. If you're eating habits are not that bad this will be relatively easy, but if you live on junk food, then you'll struggle. For example, to prepare yourself for adopting the alkaline diet, you may gradually start to increase the quantity of plant-based foods in your meals.

Another way of tricking your body into eating healthy foods is a method called "crowding out". It's very simple, instead of giving up on unhealthy foods; you simply add healthy foods to your diet.

For example, you eat meat but you also have a big salad with every meal. Or, you first eat healthy foods and then unhealthy ones, e.g., you first eat your veggies, and only then you fill your plate with meat or dairy. The idea is that by the time you start eating meat, you already feel full which means you will eat less meat than you would have otherwise. Or, if you have a sweet tooth and can't give up desserts, first have some fruits and only then have a piece of cake. Ideally, as fruits are full of fiber, they will easily fill you up so you won't have space for pudding.

*What are the benefits of crowding out? They boil down to this:*

– **Nutrients**

Your body will get all the nutrients it needs from the healthy foods (those you eat first) even if your diet is generally unhealthy.

– **Food preferences**

The more you eat healthy foods, the greater the chance you'll get used to them and hopefully start preferring them to unhealthy foods.

– **Cravings**

If your main problem with following a healthy diet is craving for unhealthy foods, you should know that craving usually means you lack certain nutrients.

So, if you eat nutrient-dense foods, chances are you will get all the nutrients you need and will stop craving.

Dr. Colleen Huber, the founder of *Nature Works Best Medical Clinic,* believes we should take cravings seriously. According to her, cravings are a sign of mild malnutrition. This phenomenon is wide-spread even in developed countries. However, cravings are easy to cure if you replace the foods you crave with nutritious foods. For example:

- If you crave **chocolate**, what you need is magnesium and you can get it from raw nuts, seeds, and fruits

- If you crave **bread**, what you need is nitrogen which can be found in nuts.

- If you crave **simple carbs** such as bread and pasta, what your body needs is the amino acid tryptophan. This acid is essential for the production of the "feel-good" hormone *serotonin*. So, if you are often in a bad mood, you may be subconsciously trying to cheer yourself up by craving high-carb foods.

To make the transition to a healthy diet easier, take a lot of liquids, eg water, herbal teas, soups, etc. These are not only filling and will help you feel full even if you are hungry but will make it easier to keep your organs hydrated.

# THE 30 STEP DR. SEBI ALKALINE DIET TRANSITION ACTION PLAN FOR BEGINNERS

## Below are 30 Powerful and Practical Steps to Build Motivation, stick to the Dr. Sebi Diet, Achieve Success and Change Your Life

The Dr. Sebi Alkaline Diet is a diet like no other. It combines the power of alkaline foods with the unique benefits of electric herbs. The Dr. Sebi Alkaline Diet provide people with an effective way to heal from diseases, lose weight and improve health. As I look deeper into the Dr. Sebi Alkaline Diet, however, there are some few reasons for failure when starting the diet.

There appears to be a wide gap between what people think they need to do (influenced by what conventional medicine says) versus what Dr. Sebi says is best for them. Some common myths like "dirt, genetics and hormones are the only reason we get sick", "you will lose weight as long as you are you eat less carbs", and "detox and cleanse don't matter" are propagated on a daily basis by ignorant diet enthusiasts, but these misconceptions only cause more confusion and frustration — especially if you are new to this dietary way of life.

This is why we have put together this **Concise Action Plan** with the most important tips for successful transition from the standard acidic American diet to the healthy Dr. Sebi Alkaline Diet. With these, we hope to give you practical strategies so you can use and implement to get the results you want.

**ACTION PLAN 1**: *Declutter Your Pantry Shelves and Refrigerator Before Starting Out on the Dr. Sebi Alkaline Diet.*

This will limit cheating to a very large extent and also keep you on track the Dr. Sebi Alkaline Diet. This is easy to do, and you can begin from your pantry and extend towards your refrigerator. Because of how easy it is to binge on junk and acidic foods, it is better to get rid of them.

**ACTION PLAN 2**: *Replace all Processed foods with Only Approved alternatives.*

Replace acidic and processed foods such as sugary items, junk foods, meats and easy carbs with Dr. Sebi Alkaline Diet-rich food ingredients (Please refer to the Nutritional Food list guide).

It's not as easy to do this when starting out but there are virtually alkaline alternatives for every acidic unapproved ingredient you can think of. So, relax and do not think you're really missing out on anything special. More so, the variety of recipes you can achieve with Dr. Sebi approved ingredients are limitless.

**ACTION PLAN 3**: *Keep it Simple*

The Dr. Sebi Alkaline diet for you as a beginner doesn't need to be complicated with too-expensive, difficult-to-source ingredients or too-elaborate instructions. You may find that getting to start the Dr. Sebi Alkaline diet this way quickly kills motivation and enthusiasm.

Nothing beats simplicity on the Dr. Sebi Alkaline diet and indeed dieting overall. Do not spend too much on expensive produce in a bid to make it enticing with different variety; all you need is simple sources of approved foods. Although, getting quinoa flour or alkaline milk alternatives can be quite expensive when compared to regular white flour, but sometimes there is a little price to pay for health.

**ACTION PLAN 4**: *Buy Some Functional (not necessarily sophisticated) Kitchen equipment and tools*

As stated earlier in the book: "*DR. SEBI: The Cookbook*", that is, if you don't already have them. Cooking with them will make preparing Dr. Sebi Alkaline Diet meals easier for you.

**ACTION PLAN 5**: *When hungry, eat mostly nutrient-dense and fiber-rich foods because of how satiating they are.*

The primary reason why the Dr. Sebi Alkaline Diet is so effective for health is that it follows the principle of nature and natural eating better than any other. As a result, people who follow the Dr. Sebi Alkaline Diet feel more satisfied than ever before on fewer portions of meals. This also indirectly aid in weight loss as it's so easy to lose weight and burn excess fat on this diet.

ACTION PLAN 6: *Be Vigilant about your Food Choices*

To have better control of your nutrition and diet, you must be vigilant about your food choices. You may find that you may be tempted to eat some of your old favorite foods, which will inadvertently stall your transition or even make you lose motivation. You must be very disciplined about this.

If you feel this may be very difficult for you to achieve, start gradually. Maybe start with two portions of your old favorites, and gradually reduce to one per day, until you're able to go a full day with it. And then, proceed further to 3 days and a week. I notice its easier transitioning this way than stopping abruptly.

Also, watch out for foods that may be termed organic", yet treated with a whole load of pesticides and other chemical agents. Even healthy alkaline fruits and vegetables are treated with these, but don't get discouraged — there is plenty of organic food produce you can get at international markets.

ACTION PLAN 7: *Join a Social Group of Like-minded Dr. Sebi Alkaline Dieters and Enthusiasts*

One of the most overlooked tips is to take advantage of social support. When you have like-minded people to share your struggles, questions, concerns, and accomplishments with, it will be much easier for you to stay on the diet and get the results you want.

It helps to get involved in online Dr. Sebi Alkaline Diet communities on Facebook or Instagram, or local groups near you. In fact, find yourself a Dr. Sebi Alkaline diet mate, especially one who is very enthusiastic about the diet, or knows the local farmers markets and how to source approved alkaline grocery items easily.

**ACTION PLAN 8**: *Structure your Dr. Sebi Alkaline Diet lifestyle and diet into a Challenge*

One of the greatest problems with many dietary programs is that they are too complicated and difficult to start. A way to mitigate this is to structure your Dr. Sebi Alkaline Diet lifestyle and diet menu into a challenge when starting out. Depending on your goals, it could be a 10-day challenge, 21-day, 28 day or 90-day challenge. This makes Dr. Sebi Alkaline Diet very easy to follow, track and stick with.

**ACTION PLAN 9**: *Prepare for the Beginner's Flu and Other Dr. Sebi Alkaline Diet Concerns*

Going from an acidic processed diet to the Dr. Sebi Alkaline Diet will cause many changes throughout your body that may not feel too good at first. The first phenomenon that will occur if you begin with the detox is a rapid loss of water and minerals like sodium. And this can happen especially by frequent stooling, urination, and excessive sweating/perspiration. As a result, many people who start the Dr. Sebi alkaline diet will experience flu-like symptoms during their first few days of the dieting.

**ACTION PLAN 10**: *Limit Sugary and Junk food Cravings with Dr. Sebi Alkaline Diet-friendly baked and fried food recipes*

You can also make plenty of Dr. Sebi Alkaline Diet-friendly baked and fried foods with approved alkaline ingredients like spelt, teff or quinoa flour, and other ingredients.

**ACTION PLAN 11**: *Consciously Track your Dietary intake and Progress with an App*

One of the best ways to track what you are eating is by using a tracking app. You can also track you weight loss with a scale. By using both, you will be much more accurate in knowing what you are consuming and have all the info you need to consistently maintain and improve it.

When it comes to tracking your food choices, you can use popular apps like **MyFitnessPal**.

**ACTION PLAN 12**: *Use a Food Scale to Increase Tracking.*

Another way to increase the accuracy of your food intake tracking is by using a food scale. Most people measure the amount of food they eat by simply guesstimating – which makes you to eat more than you need.

**ACTION PLAN 13**: *Plan your Meals Ahead of Time.*

Following a plan is a great way to stay on track and prevent you from succumbing to other food temptations. Make sure you have snacks, pre-made meals, and/or Dr. Sebi Alkaline Diet-friendly options at restaurants you can rely on. If you are at home, make sure you follow a plan that gives you what you need and nothing more.

So, try to have lots of favorite approved fruits handy and in the refrigerator. You can also meal prep some easy Sebian-friendly snacks with approved ingredients and store in the refrigerator. It is better to binge on these than on cheat foods.

**ACTION PLAN 14**: *Have Lots of Dr. Sebi Alkaline Diet Snacks Packed for Travel and on the go*

We cannot overlook how much our environment influence what we eat or how much we eat. Even with a scale, an app, and a calculator, it is still possible to cheat — especially when you are traveling or have easily accessible "cheat" foods in your house.

**ACTION PLAN 15**: *Have Only Dr. Sebi Alkaline Diet-friendly food in your house*

When we are hungry, it suddenly becomes so much easier to convince us to cheat on our diets and our goals. Hunger is a strong motivator, but it is irrational and doesn't care about your "rules". For this reason, it is best to plan for the worst. Throw all acidic and conventionally processed foods in the trash (or hide them in a hard to access place) and make sure the healthiest Dr. Sebi Alkaline foods are most easily accessible. If you are still struggling with overeating alkaline foods, then make sure you only have foods that require some preparation and effort before eating. This will make eating much less attractive.

**ACTION PLAN 16**: *Avoid Acidic Convenient foods that you can Easily Binge on.*

If a food is convenient and tasty, you will be much more inclined to eat more of it. For example, I can eat a ridiculously unhealthy amount of ice cream when I know it's in the freezer waiting for me. This is why I only make one serving at a time and stick to enjoying that alone, if I needed to cheat. The thought of making another batch is such a turn off after I finish my normal serving. This also goes for Dr. Sebi Alkaline diet baked foods as well. If you find you can eat a lot of something without stopping, you must make it much harder for yourself so you won't consume too much of it.

**ACTION PLAN 17**: *Only eat the Foods that You Measure and Track.*

Don't stray away from your goals too far by adding ingredients that you don't need, especially with spices and condiments. Adding a little extra unapproved oil, meat, cheese, etc. to each meal will add up to the point where you end up back where you began.

**ACTION PLAN 18**: *The Dr. Sebi Alkaline Diet Adjustments for Special Cases*

People with familial hypercholesterolemia, hypothyroidism, and/or adrenal issues, for example, usually don't fare well at the beginning with Dr. Sebi sea moss and some herbs. There are also other groups of people, like those who are pregnant, breastfeeding, or had their gallbladder removed, that may take extra caution before starting the Dr. Sebi Alkaline Diet.

ACTION PLAN 19: ***If you are pregnant or breastfeeding, Eat micronutrient dense foods every day.***

During early pregnancy and prior to conception, alkaline foods high in folate, such as leafy greens, are essential. But also necessary is Vitamin D (from food and sunlight), iodine (high in sea moss), and DHA.

ACTION PLAN 20: ***Follow a Budget***

Many people argue that dieting on the Dr. Sebi Alkaline Diet may be too expensive, but this is not entirely true. Although, there may be some pricey alkaline food ingredients like soursops, alkaline flours or sea moss, in fact, it is possible to have a full days' worth of alkaline diet meals for less than $3 (including breakfast, lunch, and dinner)

We show you how to do this in our shopping list and budget breakdown for four weeks in our book: "***Dr. Sebi Alkaline Diet Meal Prep Cookbook***".

In addition to that, we offer strategies on how to follow the Dr. Sebi Alkaline Diet on a budget. By using the tips and strategies outlined in the book, you can reduce the cost of your meals to around $1 per meal!

So, you will be able to cut your costs and stay on track the Dr. Sebi Alkaline diet without breaking the bank. In most cases, the Dr. Sebi Alkaline Diet will end up being less expensive than what you were probably doing before on the old processed diet.

ACTION PLAN 21: ***Use a Meal Plan That Does Most of the Work for You***

If you are feeling overwhelmed with all of this info, then following a meal plan may be the best way to simplify the Dr. Sebi Alkaline Diet for you.

In our book, we have a 4 Week Meal Plan for you to try. Check them out in our book: "***The Dr. Sebi Diet Cookbook 2021***".

ACTION PLAN 22: *Combine the Dr. Sebi Diet with Intermittent Fasting*

If weight loss is your ultimate goal, then you may want to combine Dr. Sebi Alkaline diet with intermittent fasting. Since Dr. Sebi Alkaline Diet has been proven to reduce hunger, it makes more sense and works great with intermittent fasting.

ACTION PLAN 23: *Keep a Nice-Looking Water bottle at All times*

Have a very nice-looking water bottle close to you all the time for easy access - and of course, as a reminder! However, while drinking enough spring water and staying hydrated, make sure you urinate whenever you feel the need to do so. But learn to stop drinking too much especially before you go out or before bed time.

ACTION PLAN 24: *Take more water or key lime (or fruit-infused) water anytime you have cravings.*

You can take varied amounts of iced spring water also. Alkaline water made from key limes also helps. Always keep in mind that occasionally, you may be tempted to cheat, but understanding this and getting prepared for it will make things a whole lot easier for you.

ACTION PLAN 25: *It May Help to Keep a Cheat Day*

Although you may need to be vigilant and track your food intake, it also makes small sense to keep a cheat day. Make it look like it's a day you look forward to and that helps with discipline as you look forward to the day. Otherwise, you may be setting up yourself for a hard time trying to follow through.

Many people advocate having a "cheat day". While it is understandable to do so as a beginner, I recommend limiting it to not more than the first few months (maybe 3 months). Once your body gets accustomed to the dietary lifestyle, then it's easier to go months and even years without missing your old lifestyle. Another alternative is to try going overboard your alkaline foods once or twice a week for the first two months; and thereafter, adjusting accordingly.

## ACTION PLAN 26: *Keep Your Focus on Your Goals*

The Dr. Sebi Alkaline Diet is very enjoyable if you make it to be so, but always keep your focus on your specific goals – be it weight loss, health improvement, disease management, etc. Having a constant reminder about this keeps your motivation going.  So, when the distractions come, you're better positioned to recognize and handle it.

## ACTION PLAN 27: *Include healthy fats in your Dr. Sebi Alkaline Diet*

Ensure you include healthy fats in your Dr. Sebi Alkaline Diet. It's not just enough to consume fats – but rather, very healthy fats approved in the Nutritional guide. Also, keep in mind there are specific fats and oils not recommended to be heated by Dr. Sebi. In this regard, coconut oil and olive oil are not to be heated. If you must fry, use grapeseed or avocado oil. Remember, unhealthy fats from other sources can cause more harm than good – and can counteract any good or benefit the Dr. Sebi Alkaline Diet would have otherwise given you.

## ACTION PLAN 28: *Exercise Outdoor and Get Some Sunshine*

It also helps to exercise or work out before a meal rather than after. I see many people in the community downplay the importance of exercise and workouts but we often forget that exercise (as well as sunshine) is just as important as diet. All these work in sync for a healthy functioning body.

Besides, exercise offers a whole range of health benefits especially on the mental and psychological level. So, do you want to feel motivated to stick to the diet? Do you want to keep a positive mindset and mood? Go out and work out!

## ACTION PLAN 29: *Inform Family and Friends*

Let your family and friends know of your dietary lifestyle and choices, so they don't bug you into eating other foods at events or when you're with them on a family dinner. And I'm sure they'll respect that. In fact, with such open knowledge, you may offer to hand them a vegan barbecue treat or make some nice approved vegan nice cream or cakes. And I'm sure you know that means!

## ACTION PLAN 30: *Finally, Introduce One Tip at a Time and Measure Progress.*

This would enable you track and follow through and determine possible areas for change if need be. If you introduce too many tips at the same time, it would be difficult to know the best tips that work best for you. And again, doing otherwise may hamper your overall success. Also. you don't want to do too many things at the same time that may overwhelm your body. Remember, the Dr. Sebi Alkaline Diet isn't just a diet but a lifestyle.

## FINAL THOUGHTS:

You can prepare a week's Dr. Sebi Alkaline Diet menu from the recipes provided in this book. Remember, when you are on the Dr. Sebi Alkaline diet, you may need to snack between meals to keep you on track and moderate hunger. There are lots of Dr. Sebi alkaline diet-friendly snacks you can try. Use your age, goals, and activity level to determine and consume the suitable portion of foods per day. In addition to moderate snacking to limit hunger and stay on track the Dr. Sebi Alkaline Diet, you should have and stick to a shopping list plan. When you do, you'll avoid the temptation of binging and eating unhealthy foods. Shop for ingredients you'll need for at least a week and plan your meals ahead of time.

Use this action plan compiled to transition into Dr. Sebi Alkaline Diet with ease. One of the best ways to be successful when you're on the Dr. Sebi Alkaline Diet is by planning your meals. It is a proven fact that when you back your motivation with proper planning, you are more likely to succeed.

# CHAPTER 6: THE EAT TO LIVE DETOX PLAN

## THE 3-STEP APPROACH TO EFFECTIVELY DETOX AND CLEANSE ON THE DR. SEBI ALKALINE-ANTI-INFLAMMATORY DIET

I'll begin by quoting our healer, Dr. Sebi who says "disease only exist in an environment that is acidic...only consistent use of natural botanical remedies will effectively cleanse and detoxify a diseased body reversing it to its intended alkaline state". For total healing and recovery, there are two (2) broad steps. These steps must be fully followed for the healing process to be accomplished to see the best results on reversing Hypertension. Our human body is electric so we must eat electric foods to keep our system in harmony with nature. Dr. Sebi says there is only but one disease – and that's the violation of the mucus membrane. Therefore, these principles cover almost all other major chronic illnesses including Diabetes and Cancer. The steps include:

1. Detox/Cleansing
2. Revitalization
3. Post-Recovery

I have added a third step because it's just as important as the previous two steps. A lot of people underestimate this third step, but the truth is, without it, you may get back into relapse. This third step is the post-recovery step or the post-revitalization step. It is basically simple but many people lack the discipline to follow through with it.

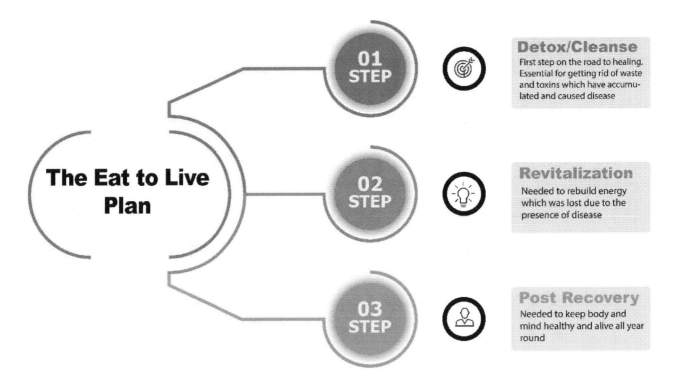

The Eat to Live Plan of Dr. Sebi

## THE DETOX/CLEANSE

### What is a detox?

*A Detox* is a form of alternative medicine procedure that seeks to rid the body of toxins which that have accumulated and that have unwanted effects on health. During detox cleanse, the body and most importantly, the digestive tract shuts down and this allows the body to focus more on healing because it's no longer using energy to aid and digestion. The amount of time that you cleanse helps a lot in the healing process, so the longer the fast, the better the results – but it is not the only factor for good results.

It's very important to cleanse at least once per year for 7 days if you are consuming an alkaline diet. However, if you are not eating an alkaline diet, you should cleanse at least every 2 to 3 months for at least 7 days.

### Types of Detox

A detox can be done in several ways. The most common is through *fasting*. They are various fasting including:

## 1. Fasting

There are several types of fasting you can choose to do and your choice will depend on several factors including the type of illness, your level of toxification and your body tolerance level. Below are the types you can choose from ranging from liquid to solid fast.

a. Water Fast
b. Liquid Fast (Juice)
c. Smoothie Fast
d. Fruit fast
e. Raw food fast (Veggies)

Dr. Sebi recommends fasting for at least 12 days on Spring water, sea moss, herbs, fruit, and alkaline juice. During the detox/Cleanse Stage, you can use the following to detox

- Herbs
- Irish sea moss
- Spring water
- Alkaline fruit juices
- Alkaline Green juices
- Alkaline smoothies
- Tamarind

**Note** that all the above must be listed in the Dr. Sebi Food list. The body must be cleansed on an intra-cellular level through detox. This will ensure each cell is purified and free from mucus and toxins. Dr. Sebi recommended total body cleanse to rid the body of disease – regardless of what type of disease since he said only one disease exists. That means, to rid the body of disease, we must cleanse all organs of the body including the liver, Kidney, Colon, gall bladder, skin and lymph glands.

# HOW TO DO A NATURAL DETOX CLEANSE

There are several ways that you can detox, but the most commonly recognized way is through fasting. There are various types of fast which include:

i.     Water fast:  In the water fast, you are expected to consume only spring water during a specified time of the detox/cleanse phase.

ii.    Liquid fast: This is basically a fast on liquids except water. Liquids such as fruit juices, veggie juices and tamarind come in handy. To juice a fruit or vegetable, simple blend up a fruit or veggie and use a juicer to extract the juice.

iii.   Fruit fast: This basically is a fast on fruits only

iv.    Raw Veggie fast: Fast on raw veggies which you'll have to consume raw

## WATER FAST

When performing the water type fast, you'll only drink spring water while taking your cleansing herbs and sea moss. Nothing else should be consumed for the duration of the fast. During the water fast, you should consume your cleansing herbs alongside and they can be taken either in tea or capsule form. Usually, it is recommended to do a detox fast for 7 to 14 days, so you can do a water fast for at least 7 days. However, note that how long you choose to do your water fast would depend a lot on your state of health, the level of toxicity in your body system and your tolerance level.

If you feel you are unable to do a water fast or maybe have any underlying health issues that may make water fast impossible or unsustainable, then you can instead choose a fruit fast or a raw veggie smoothie fast. The fruit or raw veggie fast can be taken either in juice, smoothie or whole form.

Always ensure that all fruits and veggies you choose for the fast are listed on the Dr. Sebi Nutritional guide.

## LIQUID FAST (JUICE)

Another fantastic way to fast is on liquids, also juices. Juices include all fruit and vegetable juices as well as tamarind juice. To juice a fruit or vegetable, simple blend up a fruit or veggie and use a juicer to extract the juice. Of course, while fasting on juices, you should also take your cleansing herbs alongside.

## SMOOTHIE FAST

If you choose a smoothie fast, you should only drink smoothies prepared from fruits or vegetables. So, you can do either a fruit smoothie or a vegetable smoothie. Although it is recommended to fast for 7 to 14 days, you can actually fast longer on smoothies. This is especially if your body system is able to tolerate it. However, I recommend fasting for at least 14 days even though our healer Dr, Sebi himself fasted for 90 days on tamarind juice, spring water and cleansing herbs.

## FRUIT FAST

For fruit fast, it is expected that you consume only fruits. The fruits you consume can range from a variety of high-water content to soft massed fruits listed on the Dr. Sebi Nutritional guide. Again, how long you do this type of fast would depend on your tolerance levels.

# HOW MUCH CLEANSING HERBS TO TAKE ON DETOX?

Just like every other alternative treatment, you should be mindful of the particular dosages to take when start out your detox. But one common problem with herbal remedies is the difficulty in determining the actual dosage to consume especially with raw herbs or roots. However, these have been made much easier with herbs that come in powder or granulated forms. With this, it's easier to make into herbal teas with specific ratios.

However, for full form roots and herbs, I usually recommend to research the actual dosage amount to take. For pre-made herb packages, simply follow the manufacturer's dosage instructions. If they do not come with instructions, the general rule ratio to follow is 1 teaspoon part herb to I cup (8 ounces) of spring water. You can scale this ratio to make larger volume so you can store for use.

## FOR PRE-PURCHASE CLEANSING PACKAGES

Always follow the package recommended dosage or instructions on how you should prepare or take them. Most purchased packages come with instructions on how to take them.

## FOR LEAFY PURCHASED HERBS

For leafy purchased herbs, research the particular dosage for the specific leafy herb you want to prepare.

## FOR BULK PURCHASE HERBS

If you have purchased herbs in bulk and you're making your own teas, find out what the recommended dosage is for each herb. As a general rule, you should prepare each herbal tea in a ratio of 1 teaspoon to 8 ounces of spring water.

## FOR CAPSULES

For herbs that come in capsule form, you should follow the recommended dosages for each herbal capsule.

# HOW TO PREPARE CLEANSING HERBS

Preparing your cleansing herbs would depend a lot on the form you purchased them. Although, it's easier to prepare cleansing herbs that come in powder forms, as you can easily make herbal teas with them in the specified or recommended dosage. However, for other forms form herbs especially roots or leaves, it is better to use a ratio of 1 teaspoon to 1 cup (8 oz) of spring water for each herb.

However, for easier batch preparation and storage, I recommend preparing herbs in batches of mixtures. That would mean mixing them up according to function and benefit. Again, this will depend how state of health and what minerals are most important for you. You can combine similar herbs with similar functions into a batch. Like our healer, Dr. Sebi would say, *"If you want calcium, you know where to go to (sea moss), if you want Iron, you go to Burdock, and if you want a mix of both Iron and Fluorine, you go to Lily of the Valley"*. In all, try not to mix more than 2 or 3 herbs together. Remember, these herbs are electric, and its best to preserve their organic carbon, hydrogen and oxygen nature as much as we can. Again, if you mix more than that, you may not get their accurate concentrations per ml of water, so try to limit it to 3, possibly 2.

For clearer understanding, you can use the following mix:

- Mix Colon and gallbladder cleansing herbs together
- Mix liver and kidney cleansing herbs
- Mix respiratory and mucus cleansing herbs
- Mix lymphatic and heavy-metal cleansing herbs.

Since these herbs perform a whole-body cleanse (not just colon) including the skin, eyes, colon, liver, lymphatic system and gallbladder, you can decide to choose how to combine them. Also, note that when you make larger batches of these herbs for storage, try not to make batches that last more than 7 to 14 days

## FOR PRE-PURCHASE CLEANSING PACKAGES

Please follow the recommended dosage or instructions that are provided for that cleansing package

## FOR LEAFY PURCHASED HERBS

For fresh Green leafy herbs

- Place in spring water and boil on low heat for 5 to 7 min
- For dried leafy herbs, boil longer – 10 to 15 min

## FOR DRIED GROUND (OR POWDER) HERBS

For dried ground or powder leaves or roots, mix in recommended ratios for the herb. Powder herbs are the easiest to mix in dosage proportions so you can simply follow the package instructions

## FOR CHUNKS OF DRIED ROOT HERBS

If you've purchased chunks of roots or stems, you can prepare them in the following way:

- Cut or break up chunks
- Place in spring water and boil for 15 minutes
- Let cool and serve
- Alternatively, prepare in larger batches and place in jars to store in the refrigerator.

## FOR BULK PURCHASE HERBS

If you have purchased herbs in bulk and you're making your own teas, find out what the recommended dosage is for each herb. As a general rule, you should prepare each herbal tea in a ratio of 1 teaspoon to 8 ounces of spring water.

## FOR CAPSULES

I recommend that you do research and find out what the recommended dosage is for each herbal capsule

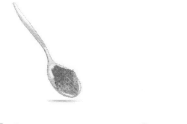

**1 teaspoon** **+** **1 Cup (8 oz)**
**Herb** **Spring water**

## HOW TO TAKE THE PREPARED CLEANSING HERBS

If you are on medication, I recommend that you take the herbs one hour before taking your meds this was actually recommended by Dr. Sebi. Your colon cleansing herbs should not be consumed for longer than 30 days because your body may become dependent on them and you want to start to reduce the dose during your last 3 to 5 days depending on how long you've been taking them.

**Routine**

- *Twice a day* –

morning and night

- *Daily Consistency* –

Try to stay consistent both in terms of timing and duration. That is, try not to skew the duration. Make it consistent and take the cleansing herb throughout the duration of the cleanse. For example, for a 14-day cleanse, the cleansing herbs can be taken twice daily, and you should take them around the same time you do take them on both mornings and evenings.

- *Gradual Wean Off* –

Just like medications, it is not the best to go cold-turkey when it comes to herbal detox. Towards the end of the duration of the cleanse, wean off your herbs by gradually reducing the dosage and/or duration. The duration of the wean will depend on the length of the fast you choose. For example, for a 1 month fast, I usually start weaning a week towards closure. For a

14 day fast, I begin weaning on day 11 or 12. You can begin the wean by reducing from twice a day to once a day. Or simply take half the dosages each for mornings and night.

It is important you do this because you need to signal to your body to begin to prepare to start functioning on its own – without dependence on the cleansing herbs. And no other way to do this than to take it slow and gradual, without bringing too much "shock" to your body.

## HOW TO BREAK A DETOX FAST?

- *Slowly reintroduce solids*:

If you are doing a water or a liquid fast, you will need to slowly reintroduce solid foods. You can begin by introducing solids like high water-content fruits. These include watermelon, apples and berries. Thereafter, you can proceed to introduce softer fruit solids like bananas and avocados. Later, you can incorporate more harder solids like veggies. All foods must be listed on the nutrition guide. However, if doing a fruit or raw veggie fast, you can break the fast right away on solid foods.

- *Drink 1-gallon spring water daily*:

Drink spring water daily together with the revitalizing herbs and sea moss.

## HOW LONG SHOULD YOU DETOX/CLEANSE?

How long you should detox depends on your state of health, that is, your body's level of toxification (the less healthy you are, the more toxic your body is) and tolerance level. Typically, it is recommended to fast for 7-14 days but Dr. Sebi recommends a minimum of at least a 12 day fast. Dr. Sebi himself fasted for 90 days to cure himself of diabetes, asthma, and impotency. It is great to cleanse at least once a year for 7 days if you consume an alkaline diet. If you are not consuming an alkaline diet, then you should cleanse/detox every 3 months

I personally fasted for 14 days and I would recommend fasting for between 14 days and 1 month if you have high blood pressure. Again, your body's tolerance level will ultimately determine the length so, watch your body and study its reaction as you begin the fast. We are all different and you may find that you are not able to handle a basic liquid fast (water or juice). In that case, you can get started with a fruit or raw vegetables fast. But make sure all foods and fruits are listed in the Dr. Sebi Nutrition Guide. Whether liquid, juice or raw food fast, the results are virtually all the same – the only major difference is in the time it takes to begin to see results. While raw food fasts take longer, liquid fasts are much faster. So do not worry, the most important thing is to stay committed and focused on whatever fasting method you choose.

## COMMON SYMPTOMS EXPECTED DURING DETOX CLEANSE

1. Cold and Flu symptoms
2. Changes in Bowel movements
3. Fatigue and Low Energy
4. Difficulty sleeping
5. Itching
6. Headaches
7. Muscle aches and pains
8. Acne. Rashes and break outs
9. Mucus expulsion (catarrh, etc.)
10. Lower blood pressure

These symptoms are only temporary and usually resolve after the first one to two weeks.

## KEY POINTS TO NOTE BEFORE GETTING STARTED

For diabetes, diet is key. Create a personalized meal plan by focusing on ELECTRIC foods that support healthy insulin production like herbs, fruits and vegetables. You must also drink at least 1 gallon of spring water daily. Below are 7 things to keep in mind when starting out the healing process:

–    *Only Electric Foods from Dr. Sebi Diet*

Fruits, and vegetables are the best natural source of fiber.

– *Healthy Low Carb/Low Starch Foods*

High Carbohydrates foods break down into glucose, so to control your blood sugar levels, you should learn to limit too much starch as much as possible and eat only healthy low carb foods in the national guide. Healthy carbs should be incorporated from low carb vegetables and fruit.

– *Healthy fats*

Healthy alkaline electric fats should be taken, e.g., avocado, coconut and olive oils, etc.

– *Limit Protein*

Diabetics should avoid all forms of animal protein, including meats, poultry, fish, and dairy.

– *Avoid Gluten found in Grains*

Diabetics can do well to avoid grains and any gluten rich food sources during the detox and revitalization phases of healing.

– *Limit Nuts and Seeds*

Diabetics should avoid nuts and seeds listed on the nutritional guide during the detox and revitalization phases as these foods might be inflammatory

## CLEANSING HERBS TO TAKE FOR DETOX

*Cascara Sagrada*

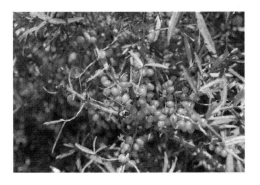

This herb creates contraction of the muscles in the intestine. This mechanism of contraction help move stool through the bowel. It has works by aiding more secretions in the Pancreas and liver.

## Prodigiosa

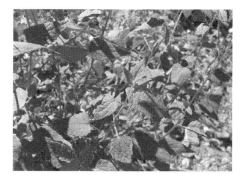

Prodigiosa helps to reduce blood sugar level, aid more secretions from the pancreas and helps in digesting fat in the gall bladder.

## Dandelion

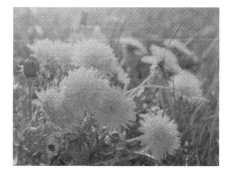

Dandelion is a very popular herb for liver and kidney cleansing. It also helps purify the blood and gall bladder. Dandelion has been shown to help dissolve kidney stones and give relief to people with urinary problems, liver and kidney disorders as well as those with type 2 Diabetes. It helps with lowering blood pressure as it provides calcium-rich compounds that helps with heart and circulatory health.

## Burdock Root

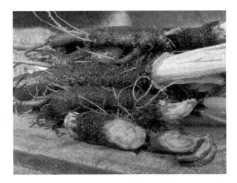

Burdock root helps to flush out toxins through the body. It cleans up the lymph and the liver and also helps in purifying the bloodstream

*Chaparral*

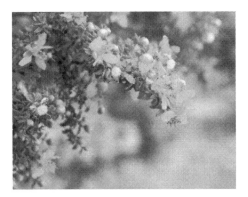

Chaparral helps to detoxify the body and colon of heavy metals and other toxins that might have accumulated overtime. They also lower blood sugar level and cleanse the gall bladder and lymph.

*Rhubard* Root

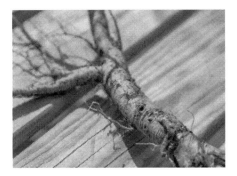

Rhubard is popular as a natural health tonic for the digestive tract. This aids in the elimination of harmful bacteria and heavy metals from the bowels. Also cleanses the blood, lowers blood pressure, and relieves discomfort from abdominal cramps, bloating and constipation.

*Elderberry*

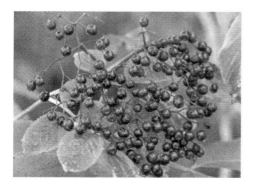

Elderberry removes mucus from the upper respiratory tract and lungs. It also helps with increased perspiration via sweating and urine flow

*Eucalyptus*

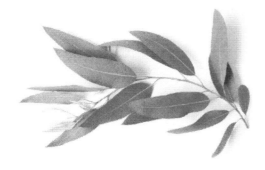

Eucalyptus is used as a great addition for steam baths which purifies the skin and body.

*Guaco*

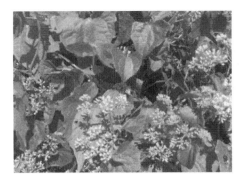

This herb helps to reduce inflammation, cleanse blood and skin by promoting perspiration and urination. It also helps to promote healthy respiratory system and immune system.

*Mullein*

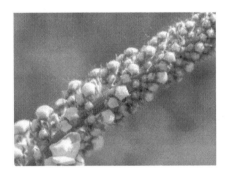

Mullein is regarded as nature's most potent lung cleanser. Used for purify the lungs and airways and has even been recommended for asthmatic patients. It cleanses the lungs by removing mucus from the upper and lower respiratory tract.

## DETOX RECIPES

If you eat a healthy plant-based diet prior to the detox, you can successfully cleanse yourself with a 3-day detox. On a strict detox regimen, most people become weak after about a week. But if your diet revolves around processed foods, you need a 2-week detox at least once a year. Water is essential during the detox because it helps eliminate waste, and most detox programs recommend 1 gallon of water a day. This is a lot of water to have in a single day, especially if your detox diet is basically fruit based. Most fruits and veggies are high in water, so, take as much water as you comfortably can but don't force yourself to drink if it starts making you sick. However, to increase the amount of water intake, try to take at least two liquid detox recipes a day. That's why smoothies and juices are so important during a detox.

# CHAPTER 8: DETOX AND FASTING ON THE DR. SEBI ALKALINE AND ANTI-INFLAMMATORY DIET

Dr. Sebi is one of the many alternative medicine practitioners who believed in the healing power of fasting. Dr. Sebi fasted for 90 days to cure himself of diabetes and although there is a mounting body of evidence that fasting could help you not only rejuvenate your body but solve many of your health problems, you need to be careful. There are many different ways of fasting and you should study this way of body cleansing carefully before trying it yourself. Basically, how you go about fasting has a lot to do with why you are doing it.

Fasting is the "*voluntary abstinence from some or all food, drink, or both, for a specific period of time*." There are various types of fast based on the definition of fasting. There are dry fasts, water fast, juice fast, and food fast. A dry fast is the extreme of all and usually denotes abstaining from all liquid and food. Other less stringent fast types include taking some form of liquids, water, or certain food types. Also, fasting can be defined by different time periods, so, depending on the time of the day a fast is carried out, we can call it alternate fast, intermittent fats, etc. However, Dr. Sebi didn't specifically recommend any time period for fasting.

## BENEFITS OF FASTING:

1. *It helps you maintain healthy blood sugar levels*

Fasting decreases insulin resistance and improves the way glucose is transported from the bloodstream to your cells. This stabilizes your blood sugar level.

2. *It helps you fight inflammation*

Inflammation is the result of an acidic diet or a toxic environment. Inflammation is also one of the leading causes of certain diseases, e.g. heart disease, cancer, multiple sclerosis, rheumatoid arthritis, etc. Even if you fast for only 12 hours a day, you can reduce inflammation so your body can start the self-healing process.

### 3. It improves your heart health

Dr. Sebi alkaline diet combined with occasional fasting is the best thing you can do for your heart. This dietary regimen will help you maintain healthy blood pressure and stabilize your triglycerides and cholesterol levels, which in turn will keep your heart healthy.

### 4. It boosts your brain function

Fasting triggers certain neurochemical changes in your brain which improve your cognitive function, increases your stress resistance, and reduces inflammation. Dr. Sebi recommended Banju for brain stimulation during fasting. It also helps treat conditions related to the central nervous system, eg depression, anxiety, insomnia, etc.

### 5. It delays aging

Numerous studies confirm that healthy lifestyle choices and occasional fasting are easy natural remedies that will increase your life span and delay aging.

Besides, fasting is the best way to cleanse your body from mucus, which, according to Dr. Sebi, is our worst enemy. Because we are all different, Dr. Sebi did not insist on one particular way of fasting but let patients choose a method that works for them.

## HOW TO GO ABOUT THE DR. SEBI FASTING

Fasting is not a new idea and has been practiced, voluntarily or out of necessity, for thousands of years. Besides, it plays a major role in many cultures and religions. There are many variations of fasting but it is basically is an abstinence from food, water or both, for a certain period of time. However, although Dr. Sebi was a great advocate of fasting, he did not insist on it because it is not suitable for everyone. Besides, Dr. Sebi also didn't prescribe how long you should fast for. If you are used to short or partial fasts, if you often diet or if you are very self-disciplined, you will probably not have a problem fasting. However, under certain conditions, depriving yourself of food can have very negative side effects so it's best not to insist on fasting if your body is giving you clear signs it's not coping.

There are many different ways of fasting and one them, the Intermittent Fasting, doesn't feel like fasting at all. On the other hand, a water fast, although very efficient in cleansing one's body from accumulated debris, is not something everyone can go through. A lot depends on your lifestyle. Besides, prolonged fasts can make you weak and dizzy so if you are in a job where you need to be alert, long fasts may not be a good idea, unless you do it when you're on leave.

## WHO SHOULD NOT FAST

A strict or prolonged fast is not something you should take lightly. It's best to study different ways of fasting as well as possible side effects before you try it. Besides, we are all different and you need to monitor how your body responds to food deprivation. Under certain conditions, e.g. pregnancy, breastfeeding, eating disorders, mental disorder, or being on chronic medications, fasting should not really be considered.

## TAKING SUPPLEMENTS ON A FAST

Dr. Sebi himself fasted for 90 days on tamarind juice (agua de tamarindo), spring water and herbs. He wasn't consuming food but was rather supplementing with his cell food compounds such as bromide plus and green food. These compounds aided by the fast helped nourish his body and heal.

Dr. Sebi's bromide plus helps to revitalize and energize the body as it contains vital minerals and nutrients while the Green Food helps to boost you fast effects by helping to cleanse the blood and strengthen the digestive, respiratory, nervous and immune system. So, both are great addition to your fasting routine to help complement your body during a fast. Also, fasting can be defined by different time periods, so, depending on the time of the day a fast is carried out, we can call it alternate fast, intermittent fats, etc. However, Dr. Sebi didn't specifically recommend any time period for fasting. This could be because everyone reacts differently, so I recommend watching your body for a few days before sticking to any kind of fast that agrees best with your system. Dr. Sebi believed it's necessary to listen to your body's inner wisdom and let it guide you. So, based on this, we recommend you understand your body and listen to it when you begin your fast. It will surely give you enough telltale signs that you can infer from.

## GETTING STARTED ON A FAST AS A BEGINNER

We advise that you begin by following the Dr. Sebi Nutritional Guide and then allow your body slowly and gently adapt to it.

For example, you can skip one meal a day until you build up gradually to going without food for a full day. Note that sticking to the Dr. Sebi's Nutritional Guide is important both during the fast and after. It's important to understand that your body undergoes many physiological changes when you fast – most especially, metabolic functions and digestion are put on hold. And your body uses all available energy for healing, cleansing, rebuilding and repair. So, when you decide to break the fast at the end of the fasting schedule, it's important to break the fast with only approved meals and nutritious foods. This will help to continue sustaining the body in optimum health. Salads, Soups and even desserts based on the nutritional guide will become helpful towards achieving sustainability and commitment towards the lifestyle. And they are highly delicious and so easy to prepare. There are so many of these curated recipes in our cookbook that you can begin to prepare after you break your fast.

## THE DR. SEBI FASTING METHODS

There are several ways that you can detox, but the most commonly recognized way is through fasting. There are five Dr. Sebi recommended methods of fasting which include:

1. Water fast

2. Juice or Liquid Fast

3. Alternative water/Juice fast

4. Smoothie Fast

5. Mono-meals

## WATER FAST

Water fast is probably one of the easiest (and cheapest) ways of ridding yourself of disease and boosting your immune system. Dr. Sebi says Water is electrical. And that giving your =self at least 3 glasses of spring water first thing in the morning could be the best ever breakfast habit you can incorporated for your health. However, you should not fast on water if you are not used to fasting. In other words, try another method of fasting first to see how your body responds to food deprivation and if you cope without major side effects, you can then try this method.

Prepare yourself for a water fast by doing a 3-day bowel cleanse. Then, switch to a plant-based diet for 7 days. Perform another 3-day bowel cleanse using only raw fruits and veggies. Do a 7-day mono fast on mango, grapes, apples or melon. Follow this with a 3-day juice fast, taking mainly green juices and the juices of citrus fruits. Now you are ready to begin your water fast.

## SPRING WATER THERAPY

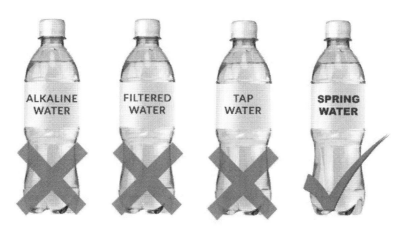

ALKALINE WATER    FILTERED WATER    TAP WATER    SPRING WATER

### Drink natural spring water only!

Water was essential for life on Earth and is essential for human life too. It represents over 70% of our body composition and plays an important role in all of our bodily functions. This is why we constantly need to replenish the water we lose through perspiration. One of the alternative medicine treatments which Dr. Sebi advocates is the water fast or spring water therapy. It is a very successful cleansing therapy that involves drinking 6 glasses of water on an empty stomach, as soon as you wake up. This should become a routine however, don't try to force yourself to drink this much water if you are not used to drinking lots of water or you might make yourself sick. Most of us drink much less water than we should. The minimum you should take a day is 2 liters although Dr. Sebi recommends 1 gallon (3.8 liters) of spring water a day.

To ease yourself into this routine, try taking 2 glasses of water as soon as you wake up for a week or so. Once you feel comfortable with this amount of liquid on an empty stomach, increase the quantity to 3 glasses, and so on. If this becomes a routine, you will drink 6 glasses of water first thing in the morning and will not even notice how much liquid you're taking.

## BENEFITS OF WATER FAST

### 1. It helps with detoxing

The reason all detoxing methods insist on increased water intake is that water makes it easier for toxins to be flushed out of the body. During a detox, toxins become dislodged from organs and tissues they had invaded. Once dislodged, toxins enter the bloodstream. Water will flush them out, however, if during a detox you don't take enough water, the toxins would simply circulate through your bloodstream and eventually inhabit another organ. So, to help your kidneys flush them out, you should take about 5 gallons of water during a detox.

### 2. It relieves constipation

Sufficient water intake aids digestion and makes your bowel movements regular and easy. So, besides preventing constipation, water therapy will also relieve you from bloating and gas. When your digestive system is cleansed, food processing and nutrient absorption become much easier.

### 3. It helps you lose weight

Water helps you lose weight by making you eat less. This happens because water easily makes you feel full, so you either postpone your meal or eat less than you normally do. When you feel a hunger pang, it is usually a sign your body needs to be rehydrated. So, next time you feel hungry, before grabbing chocolate or a snack, have a glass of water. Chances are, you will feel perfectly full. Besides, chilled water in the morning increases your metabolism by 24%.

### 4. It prevents dehydration

Many diseases are caused by dehydration, eg rheumatoid arthritis, migraine, hypertension, sinusitis, kidney stones, asthma, poor metabolism, etc. Water therapy not only energizes you; it can help you cure many of your health problems. To prevent dehydration, have a glass of water every hour or drink at least 8 glasses a day. Besides, a body that is sufficiently hydrated has increased production of new blood and muscle cell and your lymph system remains balanced. What many people don't realize is just how many common ailments are nothing more than secondary symptoms of dehydration, eg dyspepsia, angina, colitis, anemia, obesity, pulmonary tuberculosis, asthma, diabetes, uterine cancer, breast cancer, leukemia, etc. Recent studies even suggest that water therapy can cure these and other conditions very rapidly, with no other medical treatment.

To make the most of water therapy, you should have 8 glasses of water on an empty stomach. As many may find this difficult, try taking 3 glasses, have a five-minute break, then take another 3, then have another short break, and so on until you've taken all the water. If you can't cope with this, take as much as you can in the morning, and the rest during the day. However, remember that you should not take any food for at least an hour, either before or after the water. For the best results, water should be taken on an empty stomach which is why it is recommended to be taken as soon as you wake up.

## HOW TO DO A WATER FAST

When performing the water type fast, you'll only drink spring water while taking your cleansing herbs and sea moss. Nothing else should be consumed for the duration of the fast. During the water fast, you should consume your cleansing herbs alongside and they can be taken either in tea or capsule form. Usually, it is recommended to do a detox fast for 7 to 14 days, so you can do a water fast for at least 7 days. However, note that how long you choose to do your water fast would depend a lot on your state of health, the level of toxicity in your body system and your tolerance level.

I recommend a full water fast for at least 7 days to reap full benefits. Although you can do a 3 day fast if you are unable to do a 7-day water fast. If you feel you are unable to do a water fast or maybe have any underlying health issues that may make water fast impossible or unsustainable, then you can instead choose a fruit fast or a raw veggie smoothie fast. The fruit or raw veggie fast can be taken either in juice, smoothie or whole form. Always ensure that all fruits and veggies you choose for the fast are listed on the Dr. Sebi Nutritional guide. However, whether you're on water fast or fruit fast or raw veggie fast, start out by taking 2 glasses or warm spring water on waking up. In addition, take 1 glass of spring water at least every hour until 7.00 PM (or at least 3 hours before bedtime). Alternatively, you can take 2 glasses of spring water at least every other hour until 7.00 PM. Dr. Sebi recommends at least a gallon of water daily whether you're fasting or not.

## WATER AS BREAKFAST

Taking natural spring water daily on waking up is the best breakfast you could ever have. It is the best nutrition ever to give to your body in the morning. Although many people find this repelling or nauseating when they start out, once you get used to it, you'll begin to love it. Natural spring water is electrical and you should take it in the morning to prepare your colon for absorption. I usually recommend taking at least 2 glasses (16 z) of warm/tepid water on waking up. The water has to be tepid warm for additional benefits. Warm water soothes the blood vessels, and allows better digestion and hydration. It also helps to flush the colon and kidneys and improve bowel movements. I personally can testify to this. Taking spring water as breakfast alone can improve your overall fasting by up to 30%.

If you find it nauseating, you can begin by squeezing half teaspoon of key lime juice into it to for added flavor. But really, you don't need this and I still recommend taking just water alone. But if you feel you can't, then start out by flavoring with key lime juice. But once you get used it, by all means begin to take only water.

## JUICE FAST

Another fantastic way to fast is on liquids, also juices. Juices include all fruit and vegetable juices as well as tamarind juice. To juice a fruit or vegetable, simple blend up a fruit or veggie and use a juicer to extract the juice. Of course, while fasting on juices, you should also take your cleansing herbs alongside.

Start with a 3-day colon cleanse. Then, eat raw fruits and vegetables for 7 days. Start juicing by taking vegetable juices and herbal teas (as mentioned above). Take as much water as you can. Carry on for at least 21 days.

### ALTERNATIVE WATER/JUICE FAST

This is a combination of water and juice fast. Take vegetable juice in the morning, water during the day, and juice again in the evening.

## SMOOTHIE FAST

If you choose a smoothie fast, you should only drink smoothies prepared from fruits or vegetables. So, you can do either a fruit smoothie or a vegetable smoothie. Although it is recommended to fast for 7 to 14 days, you can actually fast longer on smoothies. This is especially if your body system is able to tolerate it. However, I recommend fasting for at least 14 days even though our healer Dr, Sebi himself fasted for 90 days on tamarind juice, spring water and cleansing herbs.

## MONO MEAL FAST

This fast should last for 3, 4 or 6 weeks. This method of fasting revolves around eating one type of fruit only for the duration of your fast. The best fruits to eat are grapes, mangoes, melons, oranges, apples, and pears. However, if these fruits are unavailable where you live, you can take local fruit. Try not to take very sweet fruits. To avoid getting bored with eating only one type of fruit for weeks, you can change fruits every week. So, for example, you may eat only apples during the first week, then during the second week you can eat grapes, during the third week you can take mango, etc. During the fast, drink as much water and herbal teas as you can. End the mono-meals fast with the 2-day water fast, followed by a 24-hour dry fasting. A mono meal can either be a fruit only fast or a veggie only fast, taken raw.

## HOW TO DO A MONO MEAL FAST

### FRUIT ONLY MONO FAST

For fruit fast, it is expected that you consume only fruits. The fruits you consume can range from a variety of high-water content to soft massed fruits listed on the Dr. Sebi Nutritional guide. Again, how long you do this type of fast would depend on your tolerance levels.

### VEGGIE ONLY MONO FAST

For fruit fast, it is expected that you consume only fruits. The fruits you consume can range from a variety of high-water content to soft massed fruits listed on the Dr. Sebi Nutritional guide. Again, how long you do this type of fast would depend on your tolerance levels.

## THINGS TO KEEP IN MIND DURING A FAST

- You should be urinating a lot because your kidneys are getting rid of the accumulated waste. However, if despite all the water you're taking you are not urinating a lot, take some dandelion herbal tea. These are diuretics and can be used if you notice your body holding on to fluids.

- Always start a fast with a colon cleanse

- Practice deep breathing (yogic breathing) every day

- As a rule of thumb, do not use things on the skin you wouldn't eat

- Try not to drink tap water. Dr. Sebi recommends strictly drinking spring water only

- Try not to use regular, store-bought soaps as these can irritate the skin.

# APPROVED FASTS FOR DETOX

## THE 14-DAY FAST

Two week-detox can be challenging if your normal diet is full of carbs and unhealthy fats, ie if you eat mainly junk food. However, even people who can afford healthy foods and who care about their diet, often don't have time to prepare home-made meals or are simply not interested. So, they end up buying pre-packed meals or canned food.

Not all such meals are unhealthy. However, all pre-packaged or canned foods have to be thermally processed and most of them had some flavor or color additives added. Not to mention the fact that certain foods have lost most or all of their nutrients during the production process, so to make it at least partially healthy, artificial nutrients are added.

So, a 14-day detox is not about fasting or weight loss, although depending on your current eating habits it may often feel like you're on a fast. And, while on a detox, you may lose weight even if that was not the reason you decided to detox.

A 14-day detox is slightly different from a 3-day or 7-day detox which are usually quite restrictive and very cleansing. Although you can live on juice for a few days, it may be difficult to carry on with your normal activities if you stay on this regimen for more than a week. However, this also depends on what your occupation is.

## PRINCIPLES OF THE DR. SEBI 14-DAY FAST

### 1. You must follow the detox diet to the letter

Dr. Sebi alkaline diet requires a lot of self-discipline. It is quite restrictive and you have to be highly motivated to go through with it. It is super-healthy and will help you get rid of toxins and many other health problems naturally, but is very strict so may not be suitable for everyone.

### 2. Plan your meals

Think about this diet carefully before embarking on it. Consider the YES and NO foods lists and make a plan what you are going to eat. Think about what you are going to eat if you eat out. Create a personalized 7-day meal plan.

### 3. Be mentally prepared

Detox diets are always challenging, so it will help if you mentally prepare yourself to the fact that you may often feel hungry and that you will probably have to do without your favorite foods. Make a plan how to deal with cravings as well as a crisis (if you are new to healthy eating, you're bound to struggle). Study the list of NO foods and work out which of those foods you are Not likely to miss the most. Think of what you could replace them with.

### 4. Be aware of the possible detox side effects

Most people cope well with detox although everyone experiences at least some of the symptoms, e.g. headache, irritability, etc. However, the unhealthier your diet is, the more severe symptoms you'll experience. Most of the symptoms will go away after a couple of days so try to persevere. However, if you start feeling nauseous or dizzy, stop immediately. Perhaps you should try another detox method.

### 5. Consider your overall health

If you have certain conditions, eg pregnancy, breastfeeding, digestive problems, psychological problems, or are on chronic medications talk to your medical practitioner before changing your diet and especially before trying a diet as restrictive as the Dr. Sebi detox diet.

### 6. Create a meal plan and think where to get proteins from

Create a personalized meal plan based on Dr. Sebi approved food list and make sure your new diet provides all the nutrients. With a vegan diet, the biggest challenge is where to get the protein from.

## THE 90-DAY FAST

The reason detox diets usually last for only a couple of days or a couple of weeks at the longest is because even a simple detox isn't easy and will disrupt your daily routine. And some detox methods are quite complicated and expensive and the only way you can go through with them is to focus all your time and energy on detoxing, e.g. it may require foods and supplements that are expensive or difficult to come by, it may require certain types of exercise or rigorous lifestyle change. Most people can put up with fasting for a couple of days or weeks but after that, they will start slipping or cheating.

It's better to do a 7-day fast properly than a 21-day fast where you cheat half of the time. So, although a 3-month fast could be a natural cure for serious conditions, unless you are used to fasting, you may struggle going through with it.

There are many different ways of fasting, some easier than others. However, a 90-day fast is not something you should try for fun. This is a serious matter and you should prepare yourself for it by learning as much about fasting as possible, by being aware of possible side effects and what to do under the circumstances (especially if you live alone), and by easing yourself into fasting. But, most of all, you have to be determined to go through with this.

Traditional fast is water fast where you abstain from any food and drink only water for the duration of the fast. How your body will respond depends on many things, e.g. your physical and mental health, your age, self-discipline, how determined (desperate) you are to heal yourself naturally, etc.

Although Dr. Sebi fasted for 90 days to heal himself of diabetes, if you are new to this, try to ease yourself into fasting gradually. And if your diet revolves around processed foods and is high in meat, carbs, and unhealthy fats, you need to take this slowly or you won't last even a week. So, although individual reactions may vary, this is what usually goes on during a water fast:

## BODY CHANGES TO EXPECT DURING A FAST

- During the first 2 days, your body is trying to adapt to food deprivation. This is usually the most challenging part of the fast. You feel hungry and your energy is low. As a result, you may become irritable, moody or may feel like crying.

While you're fasting, your body would need to produce sugar it needs as a source of energy, so it activates a process called gluconeogenesis in which your liver converts non-carb foods into glucose. As a result, your basal metabolic rate (BMR) becomes more efficient and uses less energy. This also lowers your heart rate and blood pressure. Most people feel drained at this stage but this will soon change. Your heart is the organ that benefits most from a fast and your cholesterol levels improve.

- From days 3-7, ketosis has set in which promotes weight loss and balanced blood sugar levels. Most people start feeling less hungry and more energetic. At this stage, your body starts using its fat stores to produce the energy it requires. You start losing weight and toxins stored in your fat can now wreak havoc in your body. However, thanks to ketosis, these toxins are safely removed from your body as fat reserves get used up for energy.

- During 8-15 days there are dramatic improvements in your mood and mental clarity. This is what those used to fasting refer to as "fasting high". By now, your body is fully adjusted to fasting. Both your mood and energy are high. You now enter the "healing mode." Free radicals are expelled and oxidative stress decreases. However, it is at this stage that many people break their fast.

- You should only attempt to fast on water beyond day 16 under the supervision of a healthcare professional. If you persevere, you should know that healing and cleansing takes place during this stage. So, the longer you fast, the better your body will cleanse and the faster you'll heal.

- Ending the fast is critical. After a long fast, you need to ease yourself into eating solid foods. For the first few days, take only fruit juices and soups, then move to cooked vegetables, and eventually salads.

- It's worth mentioning that bad breath and disrupted bowel movements are most common during the first two stages of the fast when the body is busy expelling toxins and damaged cells every time you go to the bathroom. Bad breath is normal for the duration of the fast, so don't worry about this.

# THE REVITALIZATION PHASE

This is carried out after the detox (fasting) cleanse phase. Dr. Sebi insisted that after a cleanse, you would need to revitalize your body in order to rebuild it. The body will then rebuild, and rejuvenation will take place. Dr. Sebi-approved revitalizing herbs are very energizing and this is exactly what your body needs after having been cleansed. Although a body cleanse or detox can help you rid your body of toxins and free radicals, the process carries potential adverse effects. This is why Dr. Sebi believed strengthening your immune system after depriving it of food for a certain period, was so important. Revitalization provides the nourishment you need to rejuvenate your entire body.

## HOW TO CARRY OUT REVITALIZATION

In order to revitalize your body, you have to consume lots of

    i.     sea moss

    ii.    iron and

    iii.   herbs

so as to nourish and replenish the body while strengthening the immune system. Irish moss and iron should be taken throughout the revitalization, regardless of what other herbs you take. However, the herbs recommended by Dr. Sebi for revitalization are diverse and nourish different organs of the body. What this means is that, if you have an underlying condition you are trying to address with the body cleanse or detox, asides taking the regular revitalizing herbs, you should take in addition the herbs that specifically address those specific organs or conditions (e.g. Flor de Tilla for incontinence, Shephard's Purse for kidney stones, etc.).

## WHEN TO TAKE REVITALIZING HERBS

*After cleansing for 14-30 days, it's typically recommended to start revitalization immediately. Whether you detox for one month or one week, you will benefit from a cleanse. The amount of time that you choose does greatly help in the healing process, but it is not the only factor. As mentioned before, the longer the fast, the better, however, you don't want to overdo it.*

*Whenever you choose to end your cleanse, you should start consuming the revitalization herbs. Remember to only eat foods listed on the Dr. Sebi nutrition guide. Eating acidic foods or any foods not listed can put you at a risk of relapse.*

*Also, note that sea moss and the revitalizing herbs are a necessary part of the healing process and so, you must consume them in order to restore the body naturally. You should take the herbs in addition to drinking 4 liters (1 gallon) of spring water daily*

## THE POST-REVITALIZATION PHASE AND ROUTINE

During the post detox and post revitalization stage, you should only eat Foods from Dr. Sebi Nutrition Guide – As compiled in our cookbook, "The Dr. Sebi Inspired Recipes", prepare and eat meals made only from ingredients listed in the Dr, Sebi Nutrition Guide

## DAILY ROUTINE

1. Follow the Dr. Sebi Alkaline Diet

2. Drink 1 gallon od natural spring water daily

3. Avoid table salt (Use only Sea salt)

4. Keep Grains to a minimum even alkaline grains that are listed on Dr. Sebi Nutrition Guide

5. Hypertension that is caused by underlying issues such as adrenal or thyroid or kidney issues but first be addressed from the root cause.

# THE 30-DAY PLAN TO CLEANSE AND REVITIALISE THE BODY USING DR. SEBI METHODOLOGY

When I embarked on healing for high blood pressure, I went through a 14-day detox and another 16-day revitalization period (for a total of 30 days). Below is a representation of how I used Dr. Sebi's methodology to create my routine. I'm going to share a sample menu routine you can use to speed up your detox and supercharge your body for faster healing and recovery.

I always recommend incorporate off-diet healing protocol if you want to see the best results with your detox and overall healing. That is, try to go broad and compound as many factors as you possibly could so get the most desired results you can get. This is better than just depending on your cleansing herbs or electric smoothies alone. Add other elements that support your body and help it to detox better and faster. There quite a whole lot of these things you can do and they generally cut across lifestyle habits, tips and tricks. They are inexpensive to do, might only take a bit of your time, commitments and self-discipline.

You can definitely combine them with your detox, just like I did for better results. I add ed these things to my routine and I noticed great results with mine. In fact, on the second day of my detox, I felt a tremendous change on waking up that morning. I can still remember that feeling like I was born anew.

So, I'm going to share these tips on how to achieve this and how I was able to do this and get my desired results in only 18 months.

Below are the habits I incorporated which I have added to the Weekly menu routine Plan:

*1. Drink warm spring water on waking up*

Taking natural spring water daily on waking up is the best nutrition ever to give to your body in the morning. Natural spring water is electrical and you should take it in the morning to prepare your colon for absorption. I recommend taking at least 2 glasses (16 oz) of warm water on waking up.

Warm water creates better hydration and digestion. It also soothes the blood vessels and helps to flush toxins and other waste from the kidneys. You'll also notice improved bowel movements

*2. Morning Walks (optional evening walks)*

Exercise strengthens your heart and lowers your blood pressure. If your occupation or hobbies make you move around a lot, you don't need to worry. However, if you have a sedentary job, you should take at least two hours a week and do some serious cardio exercises or walk briskly for a few kilometers.

*3. Cold and Hot Bath Rotation*

- Cold water showers twice a day (early mornings and at noon) for at least 1 minute each
- Warm showers (Not hot) late mornings and late afternoons
- Hot water showers just before retiring to bed. Sometimes I make a sauna bath in some days. You can add lavender or eucalyptus herb to the bath for more relaxing effect

I noticed quite a lot of changes just doing this alone – as soon as I finish the shower, I noticed I coughed up more mucus, and felt really relieved and relaxed. My mood improved a lot and I slept like a baby. I felt very energetic on waking up the next morning with energy I can't really explain. This is really unsurprising because if you understand detox and how it works, you'll realize that hot and cold showers help to move the lymph in our bodies and since the lymphatic system is like the sewer system of our bodies, you are ultimately activating it to begin to move waste and toxins and get rid of them. Unlike your circulatory system (blood) which has a pump (the heart) to help it pump waste from the blood, your lymphatic system does not have a pump like the heart to move the lymph fluid around so you need to pump the fluid by moving your muscles and by performing this hot and cold shower rotation. It helps to alternatively constrict and relax your body which ultimately will pump the lymphatic system and help to move these toxins.

*4. Sunshine*

Getting some amount of sunshine has numerous benefits including getting

Vitamin D needed for absorbed of calcium. It has helped me improve my mood and sleep.

## 5. Earthing (Going out barefoot)

Earthing (the art of going barefoot on soil or dirt has been proven to help with numerous body benefits including stress relief, mood elevation and mineral absorption. Dr. Sebi says our body is electrical; earthing helps with stress relief and relaxation. Think about how you feel after a day out at the beach. When our bodies get in contact with soil, it helps elevates mood.

## 6. Sleep

The importance of having a good night's sleep daily can never be over-emphasized. Good-quality sleep is essential for both your mental and physical health.

## 7. Daily Soothing Music

Music is food for the soul. And the human soul is interconnected with the physical body. In spirituality, the soul is sacrosanct. We must feed the soul. Meditation, spirituality and music are good ways to feed the soul.

# WEEKLY ROUTINE (DETOX CLEANSE)

The Detox was carried out for 2 weeks (14 days). For the first week (7 Days), I took only fruit smoothies, Sea moss, cleansing herb and 1 gallon of spring water daily. And for the following week, I ate mostly raw veggie smoothies, sea moss, cleansing herb and 1 gallon of spring water daily. Below was how my typical daily routine was for the first week. I combined mine with the 20:4-hour intermittent fasting method.

WEEK 1

Day 1 through Day 7:

| Mornings | Activity | Fast Type |
|---|---|---|
| 6.00 AM | Wake up<br><br>Drink 2 glasses (16 oz) tepid Warm Spring Water on empty stomach | Water Fast<br><br>+<br><br>Herbs<br><br>+<br><br>Sea moss |
| 6.30 AM | Do some stretches only.<br><br>Take a 30-minute walk | |
| 7.00 AM | Take another Glass of Spring water<br><br>Take a cold shower | |
| 8.00 AM | Drink 1 cup cleansing herbal tea[1] herbal | |
| 9.00 AM | Drink 1 Cup Spring Water (8 oz) | |
| 10.00 AM | Take 1 cup sea moss gel recipe[2] | |
| 11.00 AM | Get out in the Sun for 1 hour on barefoot[3] | |
| 12.00 PM | Take 1 Cup Spring water | |

| Afternoons | Activity | Fast Type |
|---|---|---|
| 12.00 PM | Take 1 Cup Spring water<br><br>Take a cold shower | Fruit Fast<br><br>+<br><br>Herbs |
| 1.00 PM | Take High Water Fruit[4] Smoothie | |
| 2.00 PM | Drink 1 Cup Spring water | |
| 3.00 PM | Take a hot shower | |
| 4.00 PM | Drink 1 Cup Spring water | |
| 5.00 PM | Take Soft Fruit[5] | |

| Time | Activity | | |
|---|---|---|---|
| 6.00 PM | Drink 1 cup cleansing herbal tea[1] | | |
| 7.00 PM | Take a hot shower | Intermittent Fast[7] | Dry Fast |
| 8.00 – 10.00 PM | | Intermittent Fast[7] | Dry Fast |
| 10.00 – 12.00 AM | Healing Sleep time zone[6] | Intermittent Fast[7] | Dry Fast |
| 12.00 – 2.00 AM | Healing Sleep time zone[6] | Intermittent Fast[7] | Dry Fast |
| 2.00 – 4.00 AM | Healing Sleep time zone[6] | Intermittent Fast[7] | Dry Fast |
| 4.00 – 6.00 AM | | | Dry Fast |
| 6.00 – 8.00 | | | Dry Fast |
| 8.00 – 10.00 AM | | | Dry Fast |
| 10.00 – 12.00 PM | | | Dry Fast |

[1]Look up cleansing herbal recipes at the end of this week section

[2]Look up sea moss gel recipe at the end of this week section

[3]Getting some amount of sunshine has numerous benefits including getting Vitamin D needed for absorbed of calcium. It has helped me improve my mood and sleep. Earthing (the art of going barefoot on soil or dirt has been proven to help with numerous body benefits including stress relief, mood elevation and mineral absorption.

[4]High water fruits include fruits with high water content such as berries, watermelon, apples, and grapes. These fruits must be listed in the Nutritional Guide

[5]Soft fruits include fruits with soft malleable mass such as burro banana, papayas, avocados, etc. These fruits must be listed in the Nutritional Guide

[6]Healing Sleep time zone refers to the time during sleep when healing is at its peak. This time is between 10.00 PM and 2.00 AM. Always try to be in bed during this time.

[7]Intermittent Fast refers to fasting between hours. It is an eating pattern where you switch between periods of eating and fasting. It basically explains when you to eat and when to fast in a day (24-hour period) or a week. There are different intermittent fasting methods which split the day into eating windows and fasting windows. It can either be a 20:4 fast (20-hour fast and 4-hour eating window); a 16:8 fast (16-hour fast and an 8-hour eating window); or a 5:2 fast (5-day fast and a 2-day eating window in a week). For the purposes of this section, a 20:4 hour fast was used.

## SEA MOSS RECIPES

### Prepping Sea Moss Gel

Take a pack of sea moss and cut into chunks. Wash and soak in spring water for 6 hours. Drain from water and place in a high-power blender. Add 2 tablespoon spring water and blend smoothly into gel (adding water as you blend).

Place in jars to be stored in the refrigerator. When needed, use for recipe

### See Moss Milk Recipe

Take out a jar of prepared sea moss gel. Add hemp milk and serve

### Sea Moss Banana recipe

Blend sea moss gel, banana and a cup of spring water in a blender. Serve

## CLEANSING HERBAL RECIPES

### Liver-Kidney Cleansing tea 1 (Dandelion and Burdock root)

Place 1 teaspoon each of dandelion and burdock roots. Boil for 10 minutes in 8 oz of spring water. Remove from heat, cover and leave for an additional 10 minutes. Drain and serve (you'll get two cups).

### Liver-Kidney Cleansing tea 2 (*Prodigiosa* and Burdock root)

Place 1 teaspoon each. Boil for 10 minutes in 8 oz of spring water. Remove from heat, cover and leave for an additional 10 minutes. Drain and serve (you'll get two cups).

### Liver-Kidney Cleansing tea 3 (Dandelion and Prodigiosa)

Place 1 teaspoon each. Boil for 10 minutes in 8 oz of spring water. Remove from heat, cover and leave for an additional 10 minutes. Drain and serve (you'll get two cups).

### Colon-Gallbladder Cleansing tea 1 (Cascara and Rhubard root)

Place 1 teaspoon each. Boil for 10 minutes in 8 oz of spring water. Remove from heat, cover and leave for an additional 10 minutes. Drain and serve (you'll get two cups).

### Colon-Gallbladder Cleansing tea 2 (Cascara and Chaparral)

Place 1 teaspoon each. Boil for 10 minutes in 8 oz of spring water. Remove from heat, cover and leave for an additional 10 minutes. Drain and serve (you'll get two cups).

## Respiratory and Mucus Cleansing tea (*Guaco*, Mullein)

Place 1 teaspoon each. Boil for 10 minutes in 8 oz of spring water. Remove from heat, cover and leave for an additional 10 minutes. Drain and serve (you'll get two cups).

## Respiratory and Mucus Cleansing tea (Elderberry Syrup)

Place 1 teaspoon each. Boil for 10 minutes in 8 oz of spring water. Remove from heat, cover and leave for an additional 10 minutes. Drain and serve (you'll get two cups).

## SMOOTHIE DETOX RECIPES

## HIGH WATER FRUIT SMOOTHIE

### Apple Cleanse Smoothie

Take two medium apples, add half a cup of spring water and blend for a couple of minutes until smooth. Serve immediately.

### Watermelon Smoothie

Cut one medium watermelon into two. Peel, deseed and cut into chunks. Blend for a couple of minutes until smooth. Serve immediately.

### Watermelon Apple Cleanse detox smoothie

Take one apple and a quarter slice of watermelon (peeled, deseeded and cut in chunks). Blend for a couple of minutes until smooth and serve immediately.

### Apple Blueberry detox smoothie

Take one Apple (cut into chunks) and a handful of Blueberries and place in a blender. Add half cup of spring water and blend until smooth.

### Mix Berry detox smoothie

Take some berries – fresh or frozen (e.g. blueberries, blackberries, raspberries, etc.). Add a frozen banana (Optional). Add a cup of spring water. Blend and use immediately.

SOFT FRUIT SMOOTHIE

Tropical Banana Cleanse smoothie

Take 2 Burro bananas. Add a cup of spring water. Blend and serve

Avocado Detox smoothie

Take one medium avocado. Add half a cup spring water. (Optional: add a handful of dates for sweetening). Blend and serve.

Avocado and Banana Cleanse smoothie

Take 1 Burro banana and half avocado. Blend and serve

RAW VEGGIE SMOOTHIES

Cucumber Only Detox smoothie

Chop 1 medium cucumber and a handful of Kale. Add some key lime juice to taste. Serve immediately.

Mix Greens Smoothie

Take a little bit of kale and amaranth green. Blend and serve immediately.

Cucumber and kale smoothie

Chop 1 medium cucumber and a handful of Kale. Add some key lime juice to taste. Serve immediately.

Cucumber and Turnip smoothie

Chop 1 medium cucumber and a medium turnip. Place in blender and add half a cup of spring water and blend until smooth. Serve immediately.

Green cleansing smoothie

Combine some cucumber, key lime juice, kale, watercress and dandelion greens. Blend until smooth.

# WEEK 2 (PART A)

Day 8 through Day 12:

| Mornings | Activity | Fast Type |
|---|---|---|
| 6.00 AM | Wake up<br><br>Drink 2 glasses (16 oz) tepid Warm Spring Water on empty stomach | Water Fast<br><br>+<br><br>Herbs<br><br>+<br><br>Sea moss |
| 6.30 AM | Do some stretches only.<br><br>Take a 30-minute walk | |
| 7.00 AM | Take another Glass of Spring water<br><br>Take a cold shower | |
| 8.00 AM | Drink 1 cup cleansing herbal tea[1] herbal | |
| 9.00 AM | Drink 1 Cup Spring Water (8 oz) | |
| 10.00 AM | Take 1 cup sea moss gel recipe[2] | |
| 11.00 AM | Get out in the Sun for 1 hour on barefoot[3] | |
| 12.00 PM | Take 1 Cup Spring water | |

| Afternoons | Activity | Fast Type |
|---|---|---|
| 12.00 PM | Take 1 Cup Spring water<br><br>Take a cold shower | Fruit Fast<br><br>+ |
| 1.00 PM | Take High Water Fruit[4] Smoothie | |
| 2.00 PM | Drink 1 Cup Spring water | |
| 3.00 PM | Take a hot shower | |

| Time | Activity | | Herbs |
|---|---|---|---|
| 4.00 PM | Drink 1 Cup Spring water | | Herbs |
| 5.00 PM | Take Soft Fruit[5] smoothie | | |
| 6.00 PM | Drink 1 cup cleansing herbal tea[1] | | |
| 7.00 PM | Take a hot shower | Intermittent Fast[7] | Dry Fast |
| 8.00 – 10.00 PM | | | |
| 10.00 – 12.00 AM | Healing Sleep time zone[6] | | |
| 12.00 – 2.00 AM | | | |
| 2.00 – 4.00 AM | | | |
| 4.00 – 6.00 AM | | | |
| 6.00 – 8.00 | | | |
| 8.00 – 10.00 AM | | | |
| 10.00 – 12.00 PM | | | |

[1]Look up cleansing herbal recipes at the end of this week section

[2]Look up sea moss gel recipe at the end of this week section

[3]Getting some amount of sunshine has numerous benefits including getting Vitamin D needed for absorbed of calcium. It has helped me improve my mood and sleep. Earthing (the art of going barefoot on soil or dirt has been proven to help with numerous body benefits including stress relief, mood elevation and mineral absorption.

[4]High water fruits include fruits with high water content such as berries, watermelon, apples, and grapes. These fruits must be listed in the Nutritional Guide

[5]Soft fruits include fruits with soft malleable mass such as burro banana, papayas, avocados, etc. These fruits must be listed in the Nutritional Guide

[6]Healing Sleep time zone refers to the time during sleep when healing is at its peak. This time is between 10.00 PM and 2.00 AM. Always try to be in bed during this time.

[7]Intermittent Fast refers to fasting between hours. It is an eating pattern where you switch between periods of eating and fasting. It basically explains when you to eat and when to fast in a day (24-hour period) or a week. There are different intermittent fasting methods which split the day into eating windows and fasting windows. It can either be a 20:4 fast (20-hour fast and 4-hour eating window); a 16:8 fast (16-hour fast and an 8-hour eating window); or a

5:2 fast (5-day fast and a 2-day eating window in a week). For the purposes of this section, a 20:4 hour fast was used.

## SEA MOSS RECIPES

### See Moss Milk Recipe

Take out a jar of prepared sea moss gel. Add hemp milk and serve

### Sea Moss Banana smoothie recipe

Blend sea moss gel, banana and a cup of spring water in a blender. Serve

## CLEANSING HERBAL RECIPES

### Elderberry Cleansing Syrup

Place 1 teaspoon each of and burdock roots. Boil for 10 minutes in 8 oz of spring water. Remove from heat, cover and leave for an additional 10 minutes. Drain and serve (you'll get two cups).

### Liver-cleansing tea 1 (Dandelion and Burdock root)

Place 1 teaspoon each. Boil for 10 minutes in 8 oz of spring water. Remove from heat, cover and leave for an additional 10 minutes. Drain and serve (you'll get two cups).

### Liver-cleansing tea 2 (Chaparral and Burdock root)

Place 1 teaspoon each. Boil for 10 minutes in 8 oz of spring water. Remove from heat, cover and leave for an additional 10 minutes. Drain and serve (you'll get two cups).

### Colon-cleansing tea 1 (Cascara and Rhubard root)

Place 1 teaspoon each. Boil for 10 minutes in 8 oz of spring water. Remove from heat, cover and leave for an additional 10 minutes. Drain and serve (you'll get two cups).

### Colon-cleansing tea 2 (Cascara and Prodigiosa)

Place 1 teaspoon each. Boil for 10 minutes in 8 oz of spring water. Remove from heat, cover and leave for an additional 10 minutes. Drain and serve (you'll get two cups).

### Kidney-cleansing tea 1 (Dandelion and Prodigiosa)

Place 1 teaspoon each. Boil for 10 minutes in 8 oz of spring water. Remove from heat, cover and leave for an additional 10 minutes. Drain and serve (you'll get two cups).

## SMOOTHIE DETOX RECIPES

## HIGH WATER FRUIT SMOOTHIE

### Apple Cleanse Smoothie

Take two medium apples, add half a cup of spring water and blend for a couple of minutes until smooth. Serve immediately.

### Watermelon Smoothie

Cut one medium watermelon into two. Peel, deseed and cut into chunks. Blend for a couple of minutes until smooth. Serve immediately.

### Watermelon Apple Cleanse detox smoothie

Take one apple and a quarter slice of watermelon (peeled, deseeded and cut in chunks). Blend for a couple of minutes until smooth and serve immediately.

### Apple Blueberry detox smoothie

Take one Apple (cut into chunks) and a handful of Blueberries and place in a blender. Add half cup of spring water and blend until smooth.

### Mix Berry detox smoothie

Take some berries – fresh or frozen (e.g. blueberries, blackberries, raspberries, etc.). Add a frozen banana (Optional). Add a cup of spring water. Blend and use immediately.

## SOFT FRUIT SMOOTHIE

### Tropical Banana Cleanse smoothie

Take 2 Burro bananas. Add a cup of spring water. Blend and serve

## Avocado Detox smoothie

Take one medium avocado. Add half a cup spring water. (Optional: add a handful of dates for sweetening). Blend and serve.

## Avocado and Banana Cleanse smoothie

Take 1 Burro banana and half avocado. Blend and serve

RAW VEGGIE SMOOTHIES

## Cucumber Only Detox smoothie

Chop 1 medium cucumber and a handful of Kale. Add some key lime juice to taste. Serve immediately.

## Mix Greens Smoothie

Take a little bit of kale and amaranth green. Blend and serve immediately.

## Cucumber and kale smoothie

Chop 1 medium cucumber and a handful of Kale. Add some key lime juice to taste. Serve immediately.

## Cucumber and Turnip smoothie

Chop 1 medium cucumber and a medium turnip. Place in blender and add half a cup of spring water and blend until smooth. Serve immediately.

## Green cleansing smoothie

Combine some cucumber, key lime juice, kale, watercress and dandelion greens. Blend until smooth.

## WEEK 2 (PART B)

### Day 12 through Day 14:

| Mornings | Activity | Fast Type |
|----------|----------|-----------|
| 6.00 AM | Wake up<br><br>Drink 2 glasses (16 oz) tepid Warm Spring Water on empty stomach | Water Fast<br><br>+<br><br>Herbs<br><br>+<br><br>Sea moss |
| 6.30 AM | Do some stretches only.<br><br>Take a 30-minute walk | |
| 7.00 AM | Take another Glass of Spring water<br><br>Take a cold shower | |
| 8.00 AM | Drink 1 cup cleansing herbal tea[1] herbal | |
| 9.00 AM | Drink 1 Cup Spring Water (8 oz) | |
| 10.00 AM | Take 1 cup sea moss gel recipe[2]<br><br>Get out in the Sun for 1 hour on barefoot[3] | |
| 11.00 AM | Take 1 Cup Spring water | |
| 12.00 PM | | |

| Afternoons | Activity | Fast Type |
|------------|----------|-----------|
| 12.00 PM | Take 1 Cup Spring water<br><br>Take a cold shower | Fruit Fast<br><br>+ |
| 1.00 PM | Take High Water Fruit[4] Smoothie | |
| 2.00 PM | Drink 1 Cup Spring water | |

| Time | Activity | | |
|---|---|---|---|
| 3.00 PM | Take a hot shower | | Herbs |
| 4.00 PM | Drink 1 Cup Spring water | | |
| 5.00 PM | Take Soft Fruit[5] | | |
| 6.00 PM | Drink 1 cup cleansing herbal tea[1] | | |
| 7.00 PM | Take a hot shower | Intermittent Fast[7] | Dry Fast |
| 8.00 – 10.00 PM | | Intermittent Fast[7] | Dry Fast |
| 10.00 – 12.00 AM | Healing Sleep time zone[6] | Intermittent Fast[7] | Dry Fast |
| 12.00 – 2.00 AM | | Intermittent Fast[7] | Dry Fast |
| 2.00 – 4.00 AM | | Intermittent Fast[7] | Dry Fast |
| 4.00 – 6.00 AM | | | Dry Fast |
| 6.00 – 8.00 | | | Dry Fast |
| 8.00 – 10.00 AM | | | Dry Fast |
| 10.00 – 12.00 PM | | | Dry Fast |

[1]Look up cleansing herbal recipes at the end of this week section

[2]Look up sea moss gel recipe at the end of this week section. You can find a whole lot of sea moss drinks, smoothies and pudding recipes in my Cookbook

[3]Getting some amount of sunshine has numerous benefits including getting Vitamin D needed for absorbed of calcium. It has helped me improve my mood and sleep. Earthing (the art of going barefoot on soil or dirt has been proven to help with numerous body benefits including stress relief, mood elevation and mineral absorption.

[4]High water fruits include fruits with high water content such as berries, watermelon, apples, and grapes. These fruits must be listed in the Nutritional Guide

[5]Soft fruits include fruits with soft malleable mass such as burro banana, papayas, avocados, etc. These fruits must be listed in the Nutritional Guide

[6]Healing Sleep time zone refers to the time during sleep when healing is at its peak. This time is between 10.00 PM and 2.00 AM. Always try to be in bed during this time.

[7]Intermittent Fast refers to fasting between hours. It is an eating pattern where you switch between periods of eating and fasting. It basically explains when you to eat and when to fast

Kerri M. Williams

in a day (24-hour period) or a week. There are different intermittent fasting methods which split the day into eating windows and fasting windows. It can either be a 20:4 fast (20-hour fast and 4-hour eating window); a 16:8 fast (16-hour fast and an 8-hour eating window); or a 5:2 fast (5-day fast and a 2-day eating window in a week). For the purposes of this section, a 20:4 hour fast was used.

## SEA MOSS RECIPES

### See Moss Milk Recipe

Take out a jar of prepared sea moss gel. Add hemp milk and serve

### Sea Moss Banana recipe

Blend sea moss gel, banana and a cup of spring water in a blender. Serve

## CLEANSING HERBAL RECIPES

### Elderberry Cleansing Syrup

Place 1 teaspoon each of and burdock roots. Boil for 10 minutes in 8 oz of spring water. Remove from heat, cover and leave for an additional 10 minutes. Drain and serve (you'll get two cups).

### Liver-cleansing tea 1 (Dandelion and Burdock root)

Place 1 teaspoon each. Boil for 10 minutes in 8 oz of spring water. Remove from heat, cover and leave for an additional 10 minutes. Drain and serve (you'll get two cups).

### Liver-cleansing tea 2 (Chaparral and Burdock root)

Place 1 teaspoon each. Boil for 10 minutes in 8 oz of spring water. Remove from heat, cover and leave for an additional 10 minutes. Drain and serve (you'll get two cups).

### Colon-cleansing tea 1 (Cascara and Rhubard root)

Place 1 teaspoon each. Boil for 10 minutes in 8 oz of spring water. Remove from heat, cover and leave for an additional 10 minutes. Drain and serve (you'll get two cups).

### Colon-cleansing tea 2 (Cascara and Prodigiosa)

Place 1 teaspoon each. Boil for 10 minutes in 8 oz of spring water. Remove from heat, cover and leave for an additional 10 minutes. Drain and serve (you'll get two cups).

### Kidney-cleansing tea 1 (Dandelion and Prodigiosa)

Place 1 teaspoon each. Boil for 10 minutes in 8 oz of spring water. Remove from heat, cover and leave for an additional 10 minutes. Drain and serve (you'll get two cups).

## SMOOTHIE DETOX RECIPES

## HIGH WATER FRUIT SMOOTHIE

### Apple Cleanse Smoothie

Take two medium apples, add half a cup of spring water and blend for a couple of minutes until smooth. Serve immediately.

### Watermelon Smoothie

Cut one medium watermelon into two. Peel, deseed and cut into chunks. Blend for a couple of minutes until smooth. Serve immediately.

### Watermelon Apple Cleanse detox smoothie

Take one apple and a quarter slice of watermelon (peeled, deseeded and cut in chunks). Blend for a couple of minutes until smooth and serve immediately.

### Apple Blueberry detox smoothie

Take one Apple (cut into chunks) and a handful of Blueberries and place in a blender. Add half cup of spring water and blend until smooth.

### Mix Berry detox smoothie

Take some berries – fresh or frozen (e.g. blueberries, blackberries, raspberries, etc.). Add a frozen banana (Optional). Add a cup of spring water. Blend and use immediately.

## SOFT FRUIT SMOOTHIE

### Tropical Banana Cleanse smoothie

Take 2 Burro bananas. Add a cup of spring water. Blend and serve

## Avocado Detox smoothie

Take one medium avocado. Add half a cup spring water. (Optional: add a handful of dates for sweetening). Blend and serve.

## Avocado and Banana Cleanse smoothie

Take 1 Burro banana and half avocado. Blend and serve

RAW VEGGIE SMOOTHIES

## Cucumber Only Detox smoothie

Chop 1 medium cucumber and a handful of Kale. Add some key lime juice to taste. Serve immediately.

## Mix Greens Smoothie

Take a little bit of kale and amaranth green. Blend and serve immediately.

## Cucumber and kale smoothie

Chop 1 medium cucumber and a handful of Kale. Add some key lime juice to taste. Serve immediately.

## Cucumber and Turnip smoothie

Chop 1 medium cucumber and a medium turnip. Place in blender and add half a cup of spring water and blend until smooth. Serve immediately.

## Green cleansing smoothie

Combine some cucumber, key lime juice, kale, watercress and dandelion greens. Blend until smooth.

# WEEKLY ROUTINE (REVITALIZATION)

WEEK 3

Day 14 through Day 30:

For the first 2 weeks (14 Days), I ate only raw fruits and veggies and 1 gallon of spring water daily. This was how my typical daily routine was for the first week. I combined mine with the 20:4-hour intermittent fasting on Dr. Sebi

| Mornings | Activity |
|---|---|
| 6.00 AM | Wake up<br><br>Drink 2 glasses (16 oz) tepid Warm Spring Water on empty stomach |
| 6.30 AM | Do some stretches only.<br><br>Take a 15-minute walk |
| 7.00 AM | Take another Glass of Spring water |
| 8.00 AM | Drink 1 cup revitalizing herbal tea[1] |
| 9.00 AM | Take Breakfast[2] |
| 10.00 AM | Take 1/2 cup Sea moss gel[3]<br><br>Get out in the Sun for 1 hour[4] |
| 11.00 AM | |
| 12.00 PM | |

| Afternoons | Activity |
|---|---|
| 12.00 PM | Take 1 Cup Spring water |

| 1.00 PM | Take Lunch[5] |
|---|---|
| 2.00 PM | Drink 1 Cup Spring water |
| 3.00 PM | |
| 4.00 PM | Drink 1 Cup Spring water |
| 5.00 PM | Take Soft Fruit (Papaya or Watermelon) |
| 6.00 PM | Drink 1 cup revitalizing herbal tea[1] |
| 7.00 PM | Take Dinner[6] |
| 8.00 – 10.00 PM | |
| 10.00 – 12.00 AM | |
| 12.00 – 2.00 AM | |
| 2.00 – 4.00 AM | Healing Bed time[7] |
| 4.00 – 6.00 AM | |
| 6.00 – 8.00 | |
| 8.00 – 10.00 AM | |
| 10.00 – 12.00 PM | |

[1]Look up cleansing herbal recipes at the end of this week section

[2]Look up easy to make Dr. Sebi Approved alkaline breakfast recipes in my cookbook

[3]Look up Alkaline Sea moss gel recipes at the end of this section. You can find a whole lot of sea moss drinks, smoothies and parfait recipes in my Cookbook

[3]Getting some amount of sunshine has numerous benefits including getting Vitamin D needed for absorbed of calcium. It has helped me improve my mood and sleep. Earthing (the art of going barefoot on soil or dirt has been proven to help with numerous body benefits including stress relief, mood elevation and mineral absorption.

[4]Morning sun exposure helps with getting vitamin D which aids in the absorption of calcium

[5]Look up easy to make Dr. Sebi Approved Alkaline Lunch recipes in my cookbook

[6]Look up easy to make Dr. Sebi Approved Alkaline Dinner recipes in my cookbook.

[7]Healing Bed time zone refers to the time during sleep when healing is at its peak. This time is between 10.00 PM and 2.00 AM. Always try to be in bed during this time.

## SEA MOSS RECIPES

### See Moss Milk Recipe

Take out a jar of prepared sea moss gel. Add hemp milk and serve

### Sea Moss Banana recipe

Blend sea moss gel, banana and a cup of spring water in a blender. Serve

## REVITALIZING HERBAL TEA RECIPES

### Revitalizing herbal tea 1 (Flor de Manita, Lily of the Valley)

Place 1 teaspoon each. Boil for 10 minutes in 8 oz of spring water. Remove from heat, cover and leave for an additional 10 minutes. Drain and serve (you'll get two cups).

### Revitalizing herbal tea 1 (Sarsaparilla root, valerian root)

Place 1 teaspoon each. Boil for 10 minutes in 8 oz of spring water. Remove from heat, cover and leave for an additional 10 minutes. Drain and serve (you'll get two cups).

### Revitalizing herbal tea 1 (Herba Del Sapo)

Place 1 teaspoon and boil for 10 minutes in 8 oz of spring water. Remove from heat, cover and leave for an additional 10 minutes. Drain and serve (you'll get two cups).

### Revitalizing herbal tea 1 (Yarrow, Lupulo)

Place 1 teaspoon each and boil for 10 minutes in 8 oz of spring water. Remove from heat, cover and leave for an additional 10 minutes. Drain and serve (you'll get two cups).

### Revitalizing herbal tea 1 (Shephard's Purse)

Place 1 teaspoon and boil for 10 minutes in 8 oz of spring water. Remove from heat, cover and leave for an additional 10 minutes. Drain and serve (you'll get two cups).

## SMOOTHIE DETOX RECIPES

## HIGH WATER FRUIT SMOOTHIE

### Apple Cleanse Smoothie

Take two medium apples, add half a cup of spring water and blend for a couple of minutes until smooth. Serve immediately.

### Watermelon Smoothie

Cut one medium watermelon into two. Peel, deseed and cut into chunks. Blend for a couple of minutes until smooth. Serve immediately.

### Watermelon Apple Cleanse detox smoothie

Take one apple and a quarter slice of watermelon (peeled, deseeded and cut in chunks). Blend for a couple of minutes until smooth and serve immediately.

### Apple Blueberry detox smoothie

Take one Apple (cut into chunks) and a handful of Blueberries and place in a blender. Add half cup of spring water and blend until smooth.

### Mix Berry detox smoothie

Take some berries – fresh or frozen (e.g. blueberries, blackberries, raspberries, etc.). Add a frozen banana (Optional). Add a cup of spring water. Blend and use immediately.

# Recipes

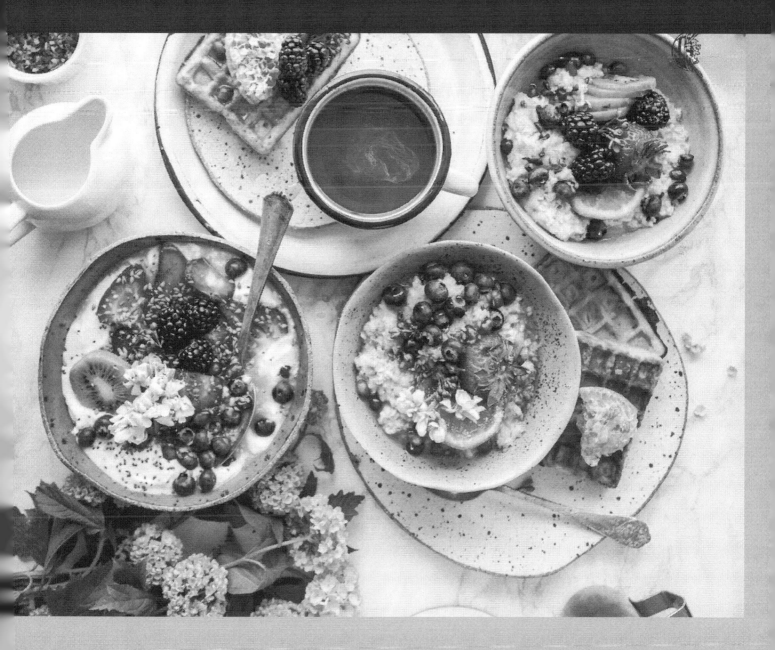

# JUICES AND DRINKS

## KEY LIMEADE

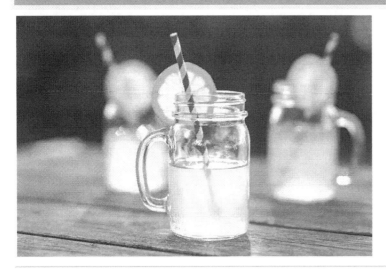

SERVING: 2; PREP TIME: 5 MINUTES; COOKING TIME: 25 MINUTES;

Nutritional Info: 99 Cal; 0.1 g Fats; 0.17 g Protein; 25.8 g Carb; 3 g Fiber;

### INGREDIENTS

- 4 key limes, juiced
- ½ cup Irish moss
- 2/3 cup date sugar
- 4 cups boiling spring water

### DIRECTIONS

- Wash the moss, place it into a medium bowl, cover with cold water and let it soak until soft.
- Rinse the moss again, place it into a medium bowl, and pour in boiling water.
- Prepare a double boiler, place the bowl containing Irish moss and then cook for 20 minutes until dissolved.
- Strain the Irish moss mixture, pour into a jug, add date sugar and key lime juice and then stir until dissolved.
- Pour the drink into two glasses and then serve.

# SPICED MOSS DRINK WITH HEMP MILK

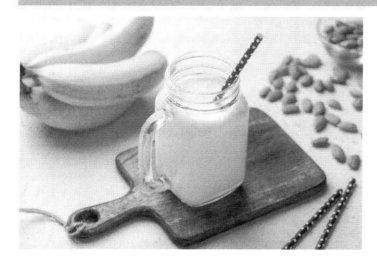

SERVING: 8

Preparation time: 10 minutes; Cooking time: 0 minutes;

Nutritional Info: 46 Cal; 2 g Fats; 1 g Protein; 7 g Carb; 1 g Fiber;

## INGREDIENTS

- 100 grams sea moss, washed
- 2 tablespoons lineseeds
- 1 teaspoon coconut extract, unsweetened
- ¼ cup agave syrup
- 1 cup hemp milk, unsweetened
- 6 cups spring water, warmed

## DIRECTIONS

- Take a large bowl, place washed sea moss in it, pour in warmed water, and then let the sea moss soak overnight until mixture turns slightly thicken.
- Drain the excess water from the sea moss bowl, place it into a blender, pulse until smooth, store in a jar, and let it chill in the refrigerator until required.
- When ready to make the drink, pour milk into a blender, add coconut extract, agave syrup, and 4 tablespoons sea moss and then pulse until smooth. Serve immediately.

# CREAMY MOSS COCONUT DRINK

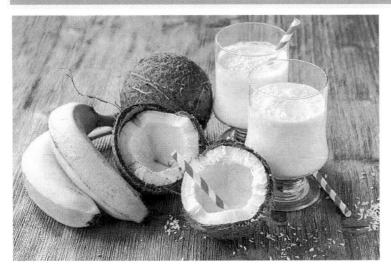

SERVING: 8; Preparation time: 10 minutes; Cooking time: 0 minutes;

Nutritional Info: 110 Cal; 3.5 g Fats; 0.5 g Protein; 18.5 g Carb; 1 g

## INGREDIENTS

- 50 grams sea moss, washed
- 2 tablespoons linseed
- ¼ cup agave syrup
- 1 teaspoon coconut extract, unsweetened
- ¼ cup walnut condensed milk
- 1 cup hemp seed milk, unsweetened
- 3 cups water, warmed

## DIRECTIONS

- Take a large bowl, place washed sea moss in it, add linseed, pour in warmed water, and then let the sea moss soak overnight until mixture turns slightly thicken.
- Drain the excess water from the sea moss bowl, place it into a blender, pulse until smooth, store in a jar, and let it chill in the refrigerator until required.
- When ready to make the drink, pour milk into a blender, add coconut extract, agave syrup, and 4 tablespoons sea moss and then pulse until smooth.

# HEMP SEA MOSS MILK

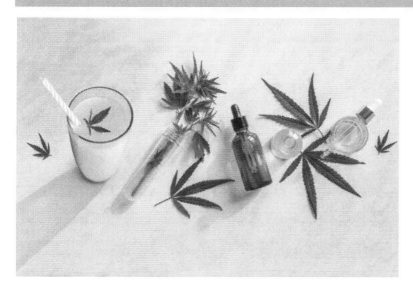

SERVING: 4

Preparation time: 10 minutes; Cooking time: 10 minutes;

Nutritional Info: 60 Cal; 4.5 g Fats; 3 g Protein; 0 g Carb; 0 g Fiber;

## INGREDIENTS

- 1 cup sea moss gel
- 1/8 teaspoon sea salt
- ¼ cup agave syrup
- ¼ teaspoon ground cloves
- 6 cups hemp milk

## DIRECTIONS

- Place all the ingredients in a blender and then pulse until smooth.
- Pour the mixture into a large pot, place it over medium heat and then cook for 3 to 5 minutes until thoroughly warm.
- Serve immediately.

# SQUASH SEA MOSS DRINK

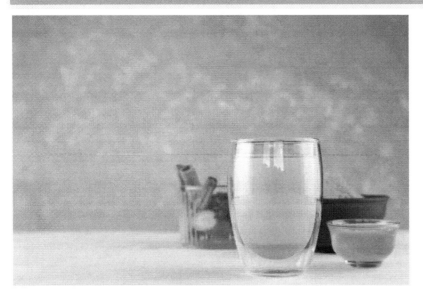

SERVING: 3

Preparation time: 5 minutes; Cooking time: 0 minutes;

Nutritional Info: 13.2 Cal; 0.3 g Fats; 0.3 g Protein; 2.4 g Carb; 0.8 g Fiber;

## INGREDIENTS

- 2 cups spring water, chilled
- 2 key limes, juiced
- ½ teaspoon ground cardamom
- 1 cup pureed squash
- ½ teaspoon ground clove
- 2 tablespoons Irish moss gel
- ½ teaspoon ground coriander
- 2 teaspoons agave syrup
- 1/8 teaspoon cayenne pepper

## DIRECTIONS

- Place all the ingredients in a blender in the order stated in the ingredients list and then pulse until smooth.
- Serve immediately.

# SMOOTHIES

## SEA MOSS BANANA SMOOTHIE

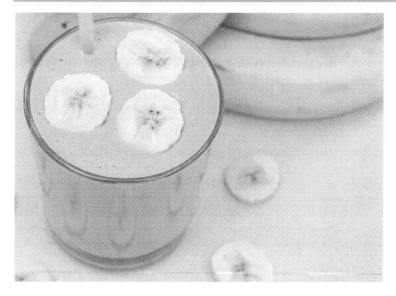

SERVING: 4

Preparation time: 5 minutes; Cooking time: 0 minutes;

Nutritional Info: 312.2 Cal; 6.3 g Fats; 6 g Protein; 64 g Carb; 11.6 g Fiber;

### INGREDIENTS

- 2 burro bananas, frozen
- 3 dates, pitted
- 1/8 teaspoon sea salt
- 3 tablespoons sea moss gel
- ¼ cup hemp seeds
- 6 ice cubes
- 2 cups water, chilled

### DIRECTIONS

- Place all the ingredients in a blender in the order stated in the ingredients list and then pulse until smooth.
- Serve immediately.

# RAISINS, RASPBERRY, AND SEA MOSS SMOOTHIE

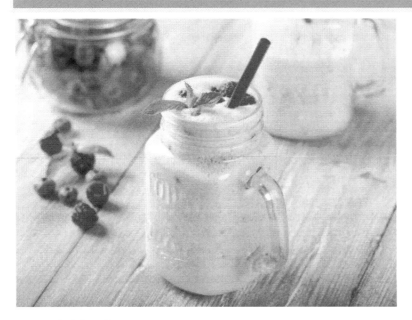

SERVING: 2

Preparation time: 5 minutes; Cooking time: 0 minutes;

Nutritional Info: 332 Cal; 15.5 g Fats; 7 g Protein; 43.2 g Carb; 16 g Fiber;

## INGREDIENTS

- 1 ½ cup walnut milk, unsweetened
- ½ of an avocado, peeled, pitted
- 3 Medjool dates, pitted
- 1 small cucumber
- 1 tablespoon linseed
- 1 ½ cup raspberries, frozen
- ¼ cup sea moss gel
- 2 tablespoons raisins
- ½ cup ice cubes

## DIRECTIONS

- Place all the ingredients in a blender in the order stated in the ingredients list and then pulse until smooth.
- Serve immediately.

# KALE AND LINSEED SMOOTHIE

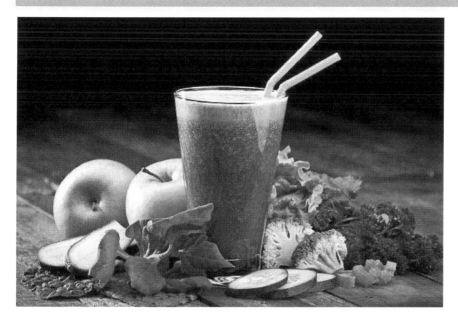

SERVING: 2

Preparation time: 5 minutes; Cooking time: 0 minutes;

Nutritional Info: 198 Cal; 2.4 g Fats; 6 g Protein; 39.6 g Carb; 8 g Fiber;

## INGREDIENTS

- 2 cups Dr. Sebi Herbal tea
- 2 cups of kale leaves, fresh
- 1 burro banana, peeled
- 1 green apple, cored
- 2 teaspoons Irish sea moss
- 2 teaspoons linseeds

## DIRECTIONS

- Place all the ingredients in a blender in the order stated in the ingredients list and then pulse until smooth.
- Serve immediately.

# SOURSOP AND SEA MOSS SMOOTHIE

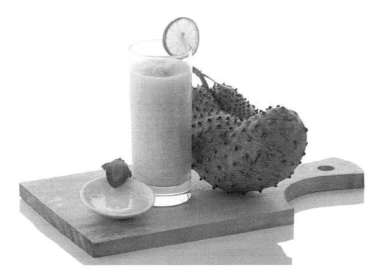

SERVING: 2

Preparation time: 5 minutes; Cooking time: 0 minutes;

Nutritional Info: 205 Cal; 18.5 g Fats; 2.5 g Protein; 10 g Carb; 2 g Fiber;

## INGREDIENTS

- 1 ½ cup water
- 4 ounces sea moss gel
- 1 cup soursop pulp, frozen
- 1 teaspoon key lime juice
- 2 ½ tablespoons agave syrup

## DIRECTIONS

- Place all the ingredients in a blender in the order stated in the ingredients list and then pulse until smooth.
- Serve immediately.

# ZUCCHINI SMOOTHIE

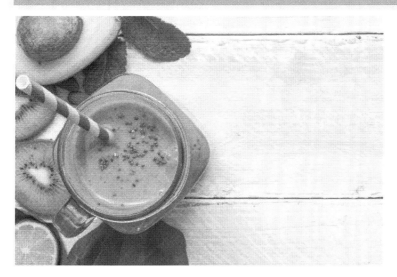

SERVING: 2

Preparation time: 5 minutes; Cooking time: 0 minutes;

Nutritional Info: 342 Cal; 17 g Fats; 12 g Protein; 44 g Carb; 7 g Fiber;

## INGREDIENTS

- 2 cups walnut milk, unsweetened
- 1 kiwi, diced
- 1 zucchini, diced
- 1 frozen mango, diced
- 2 tablespoons raisins
- 2 tablespoons sea moss gel
- 2 tablespoons hemp seeds

## DIRECTIONS

- Place all the ingredients in a blender in the order stated in the ingredients list and then pulse until smooth.
- Serve immediately.

# STRAWBERRY AND SEA MOSS SMOOTHIE

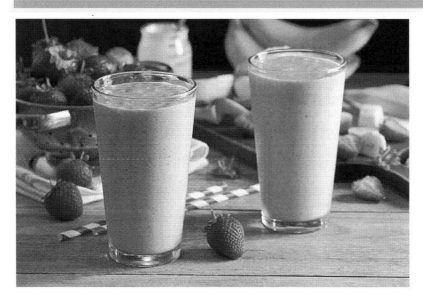

SERVING: 2

Preparation time: 5 minutes; Cooking time: 0 minutes;

Nutritional Info: 95.6 Cal; 1.4 g Fats; 2.7 g Protein; 20 g Carb; 2.8 g Fiber;

## INGREDIENTS

- 1 ½ cup water
- 1 cup frozen strawberries
- ½ cup Brazil nuts, soaked. Drained
- 1/3 cup Sea moss gel
- ½ teaspoon coconut extract, unsweetened
- 2 tablespoons date syrup

## DIRECTIONS

- Place all the ingredients in a blender in the order stated in the ingredients list and then pulse until smooth.
- Serve immediately.

# RASPBERRY AND TURNIPS SMOOTHIE

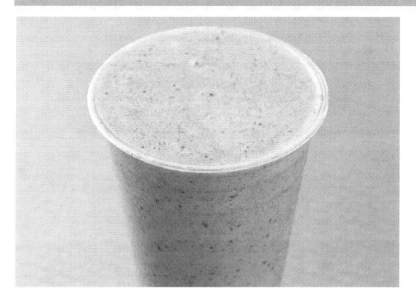

SERVING: 2

Preparation time: 5 minutes; Cooking time: 0 minutes;

Nutritional Info: 160 Cal; 5.5 g Fats; 2.4 g Protein; 24.8 g Carb; 5.8 g Fiber;

## INGREDIENTS

- 1 ½ cup soft-jelly coconut water
- 1 cup frozen raspberries
- 2 tablespoons goji berries
- 1 frozen burro banana
- 1 teaspoon coconut powder
- ½ cup turnip greens
- 1 tablespoon walnuts
- 1 tablespoon linseeds

## DIRECTIONS

- Place all the ingredients in a blender in the order stated in the ingredients list and then pulse until smooth.
- Serve immediately.

# BANANA AND WALNUT SMOOTHIE

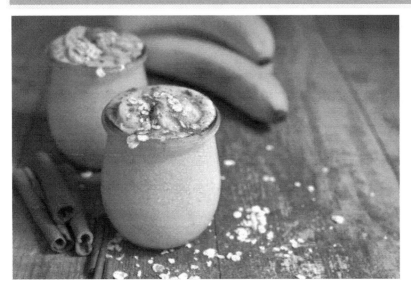

SERVING: 2

Preparation time: 5 minutes; Cooking time: 0 minutes;

Nutritional Info: 367 Cal; 3.6 g Fats; 7.2 g Protein; 78.8 g Carb; 9.8 g Fiber;

## INGREDIENTS

- 4 cups hempseed milk, unsweetened
- 1 frozen burro banana
- ½ ounce sea moss gel
- 4 Medjool dates, pitted
- 4 tablespoons walnuts
- 1/8 teaspoon sea salt
- 1 tablespoon coconut extract, unsweetened
- 1 tablespoon coconut oil

## DIRECTIONS

- Place all the ingredients in a blender in the order stated in the ingredients list and then pulse until smooth.
- Serve immediately.

# SEA MOSS SHAKE

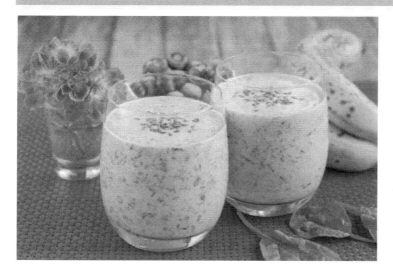

SERVING: 2; Preparation time: 5 minutes; Cooking time: 0 minutes;

Nutritional Info: 200.1 Cal; 2.7 g Fats; 12.9 g Protein; 35.6 g Carb; 6.3 g Fiber;

## INGREDIENTS

- 3 quarts spring water
- 4 ounces sea moss
- 1 cup chilled spring water
- 2 tablespoons linseed
- ¼ cup isinglass
- 1 teaspoon coconut extract, unsweetened

## DIRECTIONS

- Take a large pot, pour water in it, add linseed and isinglass, place the pot over medium-high heat, bring the mixture to a boil and then cook for 30 to 45 minutes until sea moss has cooked.
- Strain the mixture into a large bowl, let it cool completely and then pour one-fourth of the sea moss mixture into a blender.
- Add remaining ingredients, pulse until smooth, and then chill the shape for a minimum of 2 hours in the refrigerator.
- Serve immediately.

# FRUIT SMOOTHIE

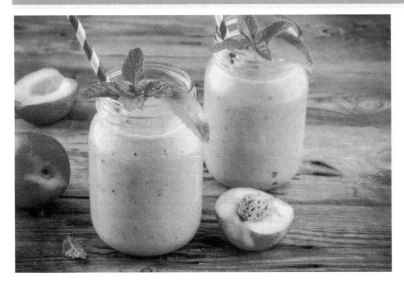

SERVING: 2; Preparation time: 5 minutes; Cooking time: 0 minutes;

Nutritional Info: 314 Cal; 6 g Fats; 6 g Protein; 64 g Carb; 11.6 g Fiber;

## INGREDIENTS

- ¼ cup soft-jelly coconut water
- 1 Seville orange, peeled
- ½ cup diced frozen mango
- ½ cup peach
- ½ cup raspberries
- ¼ cup sea moss gel
- 1 cup frozen strawberries
- 1 medium apple, cored, diced
- 2 Medjool dates, pitted
- 1 baby banana, peeled
- 2 tablespoons hemp seeds

## DIRECTIONS

- Place all the ingredients in a blender in the order stated in the ingredients list and then pulse until smooth.
- Serve immediately.

# GREEN SEA MOSS SMOOTHIE WITH KALE

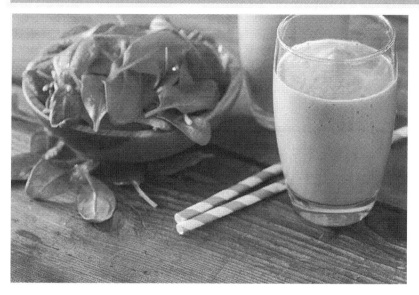

SERVING: 2

Preparation time: 5 minutes; Cooking time: 0 minutes;

Nutritional Info: 144.6 Cal; 1.7 g Fats; 5.2 g Protein; 31.1 g Carb; 4.8 g Fiber;

## INGREDIENTS

- 2 cups soft-jelly coconut milk, unsweetened
- 3 tablespoons sea moss gel
- 2 frozen burro bananas
- 1 medium green apple, cored, diced
- 1 cup kale leaves

## DIRECTIONS

- Place all the ingredients in a blender in the order stated in the ingredients list and then pulse until smooth.
- Serve immediately.

# GREEN SMOOTHIE WITH RASPBERRIES

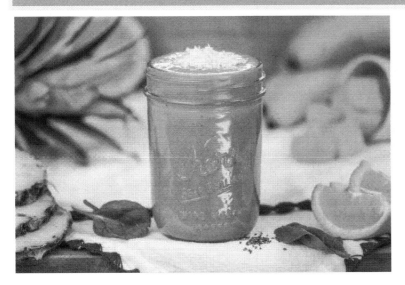

SERVING: 2

Preparation time: 5 minutes; Cooking time: 0 minutes;

Nutritional Info: 182 Cal; 0.5 g Fats; 2.4 g Protein; 47 g Carb; 7 g Fiber;

## INGREDIENTS

- 2 cups walnut milk, unsweetened
- 1 cup kale leaves
- 1 cup frozen raspberries
- ¼ cup sea moss gel
- 1 cup frozen diced mango
- 1 tablespoon moringa powder

## DIRECTIONS

- Place all the ingredients in a blender in the order stated in the ingredients list and then pulse until smooth.
- Serve immediately.

# LEAN GREEN SMOOTHIE

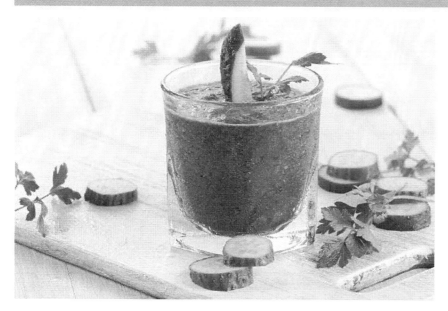

SERVING: 2

Preparation time: 5 minutes; Cooking time: 0 minutes;

Nutritional Info: 455 Cal; 18 g Fats; 17 g Protein; 63 g Carb; 9 g Fiber;

## INGREDIENTS

- 1 ½ cup soft-jelly coconut water
- 2 pears, diced
- 2 small cucumbers
- ¼ cup sea moss gel
- 1 ½ cup grapes

## DIRECTIONS

- Place all the ingredients in a blender in the order stated in the ingredients list and then pulse until smooth.
- Serve immediately.

# AVOCADO SMOOTHIE

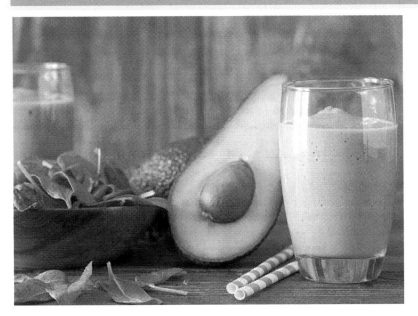

SERVING: 2

Preparation time: 5 minutes; Cooking time: 0 minutes;

Nutritional Info: 370 Cal; 21 g Fats; 8 g Protein; 44 g Carb; 11 g Fiber;

## INGREDIENTS

- 3 cups walnut milk, unsweetened
- 2 medium pears, diced
- 2 avocados, peeled, pitted,
- ¼ cup sea moss gel
- 2 teaspoons maca powder

## DIRECTIONS

- Place all the ingredients in a blender in the order stated in the ingredients list and then pulse until smooth.
- Serve immediately.

# WATERMELON SMOOTHIE

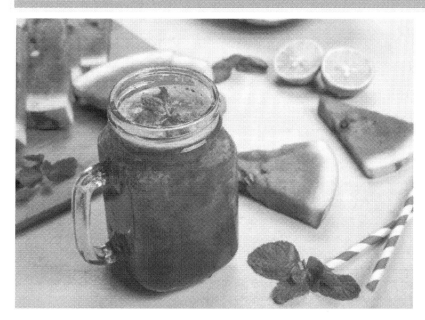

SERVING: 2

Preparation time: 5 minutes; Cooking time: 0 minutes;

Nutritional Info: 227 Cal; 3.4 g Fats; 8.6 g Protein; 44.2 g Carb; 1.8 g Fiber;

## INGREDIENTS

- 1 cup walnut milk, unsweetened
- 3 cups watermelon chunks
- 2 tablespoons raisins
- 3 tablespoons basil leaves
- 2 Medjool dates, pitted

## DIRECTIONS

- Place all the ingredients in a blender in the order stated in the ingredients list and then pulse until smooth.
- Serve immediately.

# MORNING DETOX SMOOTHIE

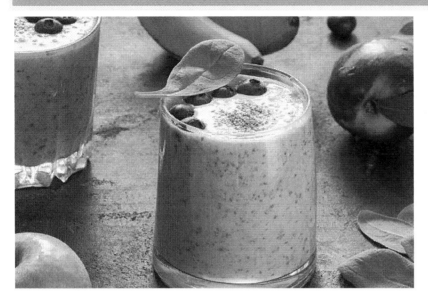

SERVING: 2

Preparation time: 5 minutes; Cooking time: 0 minutes;

Nutritional Info: 156 Cal; 4 g Fats; 3 g Protein; 30 g Carb; 4.5 g Fiber;

## INGREDIENTS

- 1 cup frozen blueberries
- 1 teaspoon Maca
- 1 cup kale leaves
- ¼ cup sea moss gel
- 1 cup lettuce leaves
- 1 tablespoon Moringa powder
- 1 tablespoon linseeds

## DIRECTIONS

- Place all the ingredients in a blender in the order stated in the ingredients list and then pulse until smooth.
- Serve immediately.

# TROPICAL PAPAYA SMOOTHIE

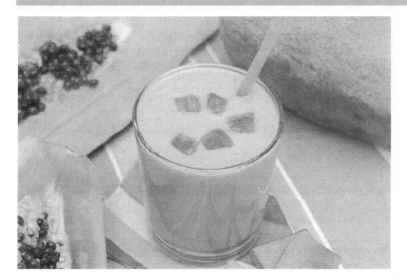

SERVING: 2

Preparation time: 5 minutes; Cooking time: 0 minutes;

Nutritional Info: 191 Cal; 3.2 g Fats; 12.6 g Protein; 31.5 g Carb; 5.8 g Fiber;

## INGREDIENTS

- 1 cup soft-jelly coconut milk, unsweetened
- ½ of large papaya, cut into cubes
- 2 Medjool dates, pitted
- 1 ½ cup frozen mango
- 3 tablespoons grated soft-jelly coconut

## DIRECTIONS

- Place all the ingredients in a blender in the order stated in the ingredients list and then pulse until smooth.
- Serve immediately.

# SOOTHING SMOOTHIE

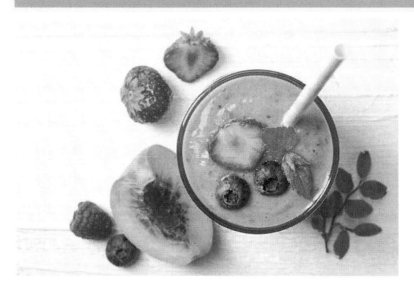

SERVING: 2

Preparation time: 5 minutes; Cooking time: 0 minutes;

Nutritional Info: 360 Cal; 6 g Fats; 11 g Protein; 75 g Carb; 18 g Fiber;

## INGREDIENTS

- 2 cups hemp milk
- ½ cup strawberries
- ½ cup blueberries
- ¼ cup sea moss
- 1 cup diced peaches
- 2 Medjool dates, pitted

## DIRECTIONS

- Place all the ingredients in a blender in the order stated in the ingredients list and then pulse until smooth.
- Serve immediately.

# DESSERTS

## BLANC-MANGE PUDDING

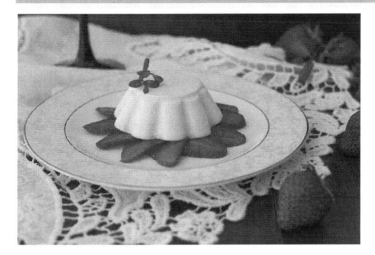

SERVING: 4; Prep time: 1 hour; Cook time: 25 minutes;

Nutritional Info: 48.4 Cal; 1.4 g Fats; 0.6 g Protein; 8.7 g Carb; 0.9 g Fiber;

### INGREDIENTS

- 12 grams dried Irish moss seaweed, rinsed
- 3 tablespoons agave
- 1 key lime, zested
- 1/8 teaspoon coconut extract, unsweetened
- 3 tablespoons chickpea water
- 2 cups soft-jelly coconut milk, unsweetened

### DIRECTIONS

- Place the rinsed moss seaweed in a small bowl, cover with warm water and then let it soak for 15 minutes.
- Then drain the moss seaweed, place it in a medium saucepan and then add coconut extract, key lime zest, and milk.
- Stir until mixed, place the saucepan over medium heat, bring to boil, and then simmer for 25 minutes until mixture begins to thicken.

- Meanwhile, take a small bowl, place chickpea water in it, add agave and then whisk until well combined.
- Strain the Irish moss mixture into it, whisking continuously, and then set aside until cooled completely.
- Place the bowl in the refrigerator for 1 hour or more until set and then serve with berries.

## WHITE FAUX CHOCOLATE PIE

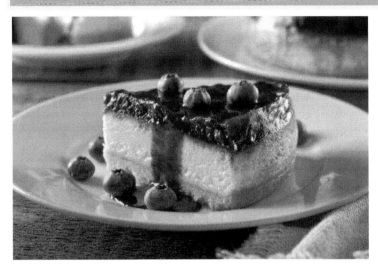

SERVING: 8; Preparation time: 7 hours and 10 minutes; Cooking time: 0 minutes;

Nutritional Info: 398 Cal; 32 g Fats; 7 g Protein; 27 g Carb; 3 g Fiber;

INGREDIENTS

For the Cake:
- 50 grams spelt flour
- 2 tablespoons lecithin
- 3 cups Irish sea moss paste
- 1 teaspoon sea salt
- 2 tablespoons coconut extract, unsweetened
- 1 cup agave syrup
- 1 cup coconut oil
  For the Topping:
- 2 tablespoons agave syrup
- 2 cups blueberries
- 2 tablespoons Irish sea moss paste

## DIRECTIONS

- Place the Irish Sea moss paste into a blender, add flour and then pulse until smooth.
- Add remaining ingredients for the cake in it, blend until well combined, spoon into a pie pan, and then spread the mixture evenly.
- Take a medium bowl, place all the ingredients for the topping in it and then blend lightly until just combined.
- Spread the topping over the cake and then refrigerate for a minimum of 7 hours until set.
- Cut the cake into slices and then serve.

# KEY LIME PARFAIT

SERVING: 6

Preparation time: 7 hours and 5 minutes; Cooking time: 0 minutes;

Nutritional Info: 500 Cal; 29 g Fats; 3 g Protein; 61 g Carb; 3 g Fiber;

## INGREDIENTS

- ½ cup key lime juice
- 2 tablespoons lecithin
- 1/8 teaspoon stevia
- 3 cups Irish sea moss paste
- ¾ teaspoon sea salt
- ¾ cup coconut oil
- 1 cup spring water

## DIRECTIONS

- Place all the ingredients in a food processor and then pulse until smooth and creamy.
- Divide the parfait evenly among 6 glasses, then refrigerate for a minimum of 7 hours and serve.

# VEGAN CARAMEL FRAPPE

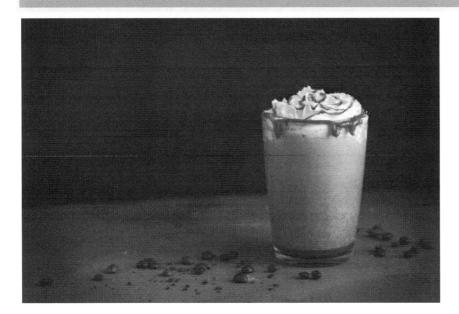

SERVING: 4

Preparation time: 5 minutes; Cooking time: 0 minutes;

Nutritional Info: 226 Cal; 6.2 g Fats; 3.8 g Protein; 40 g Carb; 6 g Fiber;

## INGREDIENTS

- ½ teaspoon Lucuma powder
- 4 tablespoons agave syrup
- 1/8 cup coconut butter, melted
- 4 cups burdock tea
- 2 tablespoons Irish sea moss paste
- 2 tablespoons coconut extract, unsweetened
- 1 tablespoon coconut oil

## DIRECTIONS

- Place all the ingredients in a food processor and then pulse until smooth and creamy.
- Divide the frappe evenly among 4 glasses and then serve.

# QUINT'S ESPRESSO PUDDING

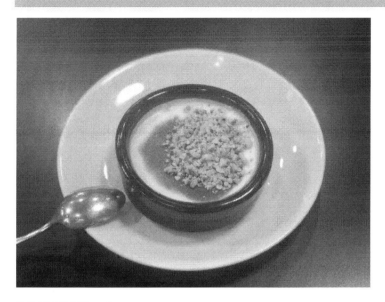

SERVING: 4

Preparation time: 2 hours and 5 minutes; Cooking time: 0 minutes;

Nutritional Info: 89.2 Cal; 1.9 g Fats; 1 g Protein; 17.7 g Carb; 1.4 g Fiber;

## INGREDIENTS

- 3 tablespoon Irish sea moss paste
- 3 tablespoons agave syrup
- 2 tablespoons coconut extract, unsweetened
- ½ teaspoon lavender powder
- ½ teaspoon coconut oil
- 1 teaspoon coconut butter, melted
- 1 dried red chili pepper
- 2 cups Cat whiskers tea

## DIRECTIONS

- Place all the ingredients in a food processor and then pulse until smooth and creamy.
- Divide the pudding evenly among 4 bowls, then refrigerate for a minimum of 2 hours until set and serve.

## STRAWBERRY AND BANANA ICE CREAM

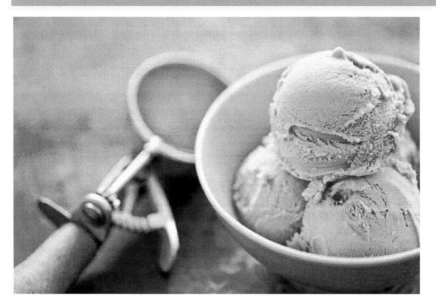

SERVING: 4

Preparation time: 10 minutes; Cooking time: 0 minutes;

Nutritional Info: 196 Cal; 1 g Fats; 2 g Protein; 49 g Carb; 5 g Fiber;

### INGREDIENTS

- 2 ½ cups chopped burro bananas, frozen
- ½ small key lime, juiced
- 1 cup strawberries, frozen
- 3 tablespoons agave syrup
- ¼ cup sea moss gel
- 2 tablespoons hemp milk

### DIRECTIONS

- Freeze the banana pieces and strawberries and then place them into a blender.
- Add remaining ingredients and then pulse until smooth.
- Divide the ice cream evenly among four bowls and then serve.

# COCONUT ICE CREAM

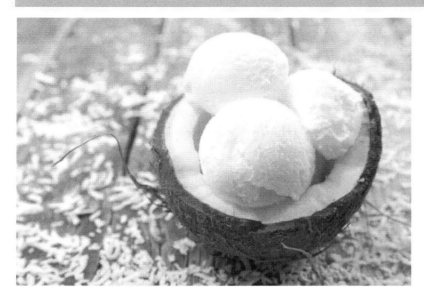

SERVING: 4

Preparation time: 4 hours and 25 minutes; Cooking time: 0 minutes;

Nutritional Info: 279 Cal; 19.8 g Fats; 2.5 g Protein; 23.9 g Carb; 2.8 g Fiber;

## INGREDIENTS

- 2 tablespoons Irish sea moss gel
- 1 tablespoon agave
- ¼ cup agave syrup
- 14 ounces coconut milk, full-fat

## DIRECTIONS

- Place all the ingredients in a blender, and then pulse until blended.
- Pour the mixture into a large bowl, cover with its lid and then let it freeze for a minimum of 4 hours until set.
- When ready to eat, thaw the ice cream for 20 minutes and then scoop into bowls.
- Serve straight away.

# PANNA COTTA

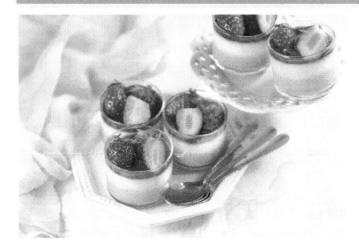

SERVING: 6; Prep time: 2 hours; Cooking time: 0 minutes;

## INGREDIENTS

- ½ cup coconut meat
- 2/3 cup-soaked walnuts
- 1/8 teaspoon sea salt
- 1 tablespoon of Bromide Plus Powder
- ¼ cup agave syrup and more as needed
- ¼ cup and 1 tablespoon coconut oil
- 2 cups and 2 tablespoons coconut water
- ½ cup strawberries, sliced

## DIRECTIONS

- Drain the walnuts, place them in a food processor, add coconut water, and then blend until very smooth.
- Strain the mixture into a bowl, return the milk into the blender, add coconut, agave syrup, and Bromide plus powder and then blend until smooth.
- Take six ramekins, grease them with coconut oil, divide the mixture evenly among them and then chill for a minimum of 2 hours until set.
- Top the panna cotta with strawberries, drizzle with some more agave syrup and then serve.

# MOCK CHOCOLATE PUDDING

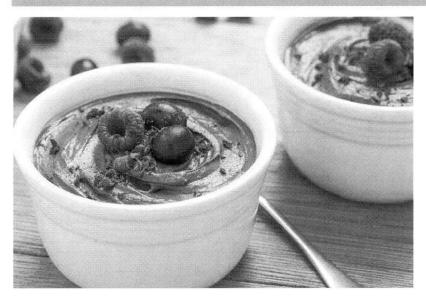

SERVING: 2

Preparation time: 3 hours and 10 minutes; Cooking time: 0 minutes;

Nutritional Info: 109.2 Cal; 2.5 g Fats; 5.1 g Protein; 19.9 g Carb; 2.9 g Fiber;

## INGREDIENTS

- 2 black sapote, seeded, mashed
- 2 teaspoons coconut extract, unsweetened
- 1/3 cup agave syrup
- 1 cup Irish sea moss gel
- ¼ cup coconut oil
- 3 cups coconut milk, unsweetened

## DIRECTIONS

- Place all the ingredients in a blender and then pulse until smooth.
- Divide the pudding evenly among six mason jars, refrigerate for a minimum of 3 hours until set and then serve.

## SQUASH PUDDING

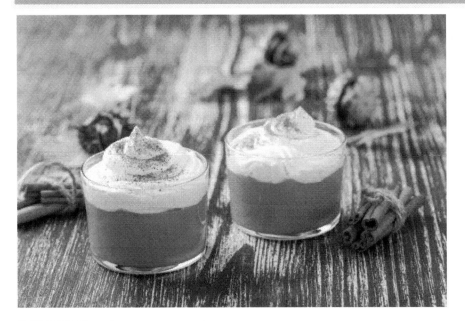

SERVING: 4

Preparation time: 5 minutes; Cooking time: 10 minutes;

Nutritional Info: 158 Cal; 2 g Fats; 3 g Protein; 33 g Carb; 2 g Fiber;

## INGREDIENTS

- 6 Medjool dates, pitted
- 2 tablespoons mesquite powder
- 1 teaspoon pumpkin pie spice
- ½ cup Irish moss gel
- 1 teaspoon coconut extract, unsweetened
- 2 tablespoons walnut butter
- 2/3 cup walnut milk
- 2 cups squash puree

## DIRECTIONS

- Place all the ingredients in a blender and then pulse until smooth.
- Divide the pudding evenly among four mason jars, refrigerate for a minimum of 3 hours until set and then serve.

# SQUASH MOUSSE PIE

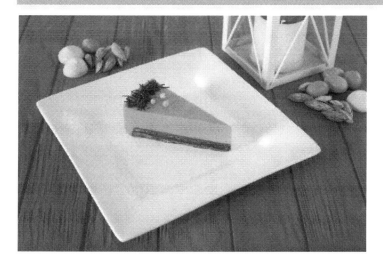

SERVING: 6; Preparation time: 2 hours and 10 minutes; Cooking time: 0 minutes;

Nutritional Info: 360 Cal; 20.6 g Fats; 4.3 g Protein; 42.4 g Carb; 3.6 g Fiber;

## INGREDIENTS

For the Mousse:
- 1 1/3 cup Brazil nuts, soaked
- 2 tablespoons Irish sea moss gel
- ¼ cup agave syrup
- 6 tablespoons coconut oil
- ¼ cup water
- 2 cups squash puree
For the Crust:
- 1/3 cup Medjool dates, pitted
- 1 cup walnuts
- 1/8 teaspoon sea salt

## DIRECTIONS

- Prepare the mousse and for this, place all of its ingredients in a blender and then pulse until smooth.
- Prepare the crust and for this, place pecans in a blender, add salt, and then pulse until a crumbled mixture comes together.

- Add dates, pulse until well combined, spoon the mixture into a pie pan, and then spread evenly in the bottom.
- Spoon the mousse over the crust, spread it evenly, and then refrigerate for a minimum of 2 hours.
- Serve immediately.

# SALADS

## RAINBOW MANGO SALAD

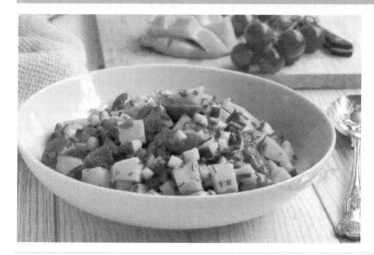

SERVING: 2

Preparation time: 10 minutes; Cooking time: 0 minutes;

Nutritional Info: 108 Cal; 0.5 g Fats; 1 g Protein; 28.1 g Carb; 3.3 g Fiber;

### INGREDIENTS

- 1 mango, peeled, destoned, cubed
- ¼ of onion, chopped
- ½ cup cherry tomatoes, halved
- ½ of cucumber, deseeded, sliced
- ½ of green bell pepper, deseeded, sliced

Extra:
- 1/3 teaspoon salt
- ¼ teaspoon cayenne pepper
- ¼ of key lime, juiced

### DIRECTIONS

1. Take a medium bowl, place the mango pieces in it, add onion, tomatoes, cucumber, and bell pepper and then drizzle with lime juice.
2. Season with salt and cayenne pepper, toss until combined, and let the salad rest in the refrigerator for a minimum of 20 minutes.
3. Serve straight away.

# SATISFYING SPRING SALAD

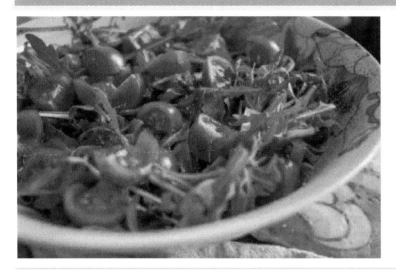

SERVING: 2

Preparation time: 5 minutes; Cooking time: 10 minutes;

Nutritional Info: 87.3 Cal; 7 g Fats; 1.4 g Protein; 6 g Carb; 1.3 g Fiber;

## INGREDIENTS

- 4 ounces arugula
- ½ cup cherry tomatoes, halved
- ¼ cup basil leaves
- ½ key lime, juiced
- 2 tablespoons walnuts

Extra:
- ¼ teaspoon salt
- 1/8 teaspoon cayenne pepper
- ½ tablespoon tahini butter

## DIRECTIONS

1. Prepare the dressing and for this, take a small bowl, place key lime juice in it, add tahini butter, salt, and cayenne pepper and then whisk until combined.
2. Take a medium bowl, place arugula, tomatoes and basil leaves in it, pour in the dressing, and then massage by using your hands.
3. Let the salad rest for 20 minutes, then taste to adjust seasoning and then serve.

# DANDELION AND STRAWBERRY SALAD

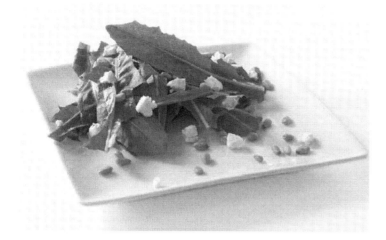

SERVING: 2

Preparation time: 10 minutes; Cooking time: 7 minutes;

Nutritional Info: 204 Cal; 16.1 g Fats; 7 g Protein; 10.6 g Carb; 2.8 g Fiber;

## INGREDIENTS

- ½ of onion, peeled, sliced
- 5 strawberries, sliced
- 2 cups dandelion greens, rinsed
- 1 tablespoon key lime juice
- 1 tablespoon grapeseed oil

Extra:
- ¼ teaspoon salt

## DIRECTIONS

1. Take a medium skillet pan, place it over medium heat, add oil and let it heat until warm.
2. Add onion, season with 1/8 teaspoon salt, stir until mixed, and then cook for 3 to 5 minutes until tender and golden brown.
3. Meanwhile, take a small bowl, place slices of strawberries in it, drizzle with ½ tablespoon lime juice and then toss until coated.
4. When onions have turned golden brown, stir in remaining lime juice, stir until mixed, and then cook for 1 minute.
5. Remove pan from heat, transfer onions into a large salad bowl, add strawberries along with their juices and dandelion greens and then sprinkle with remaining salt. Toss until mixed and then serve.

# SPICY WAKAME SALAD

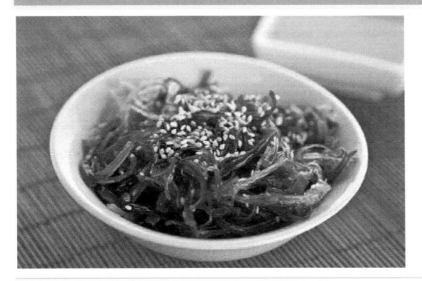

## SERVING: 2

Preparation time: 15 minutes; Cooking time: 0 minutes;

Nutritional Info: 106 Cal; 7.3 g Fats; 3 g Protein; 8 g Carb; 1.7 g Fiber;

### INGREDIENTS

- 1 cup wakame stems
- ½ tablespoon chopped red bell pepper
- ½ teaspoon onion powder
- ½ tablespoon key lime juice

Extra:
- ½ tablespoon agave syrup
- ½ tablespoon sesame seeds
- ½ tablespoon sesame oil

### DIRECTIONS

1. Place wakame stems in a bowl, cover with water, let them soak for 10 minutes, and then drain.
2. Meanwhile, prepare the dressing and for this, take a small bowl, add lime juice, onion, agave syrup and sesame oil in it and then whisk until blended.
3. Place drained wakame stems in a large dish, add bell pepper, pour in the dressing and then toss until coated.
4. Sprinkle sesame seeds over the salad and then serve.

# AVO-ORANGE SALAD DISH

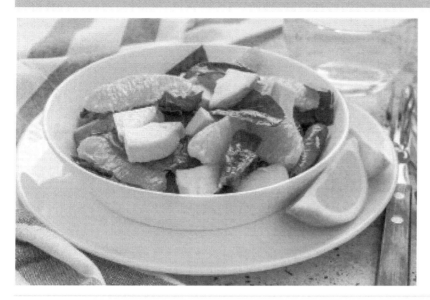

SERVING: 2

Preparation time: 5 minutes; Cooking time: 0 minutes;

Nutritional Info: 228 Cal; 18.9 g Fats; 3.3 g Protein; 14.7 g Carb; 7 g Fiber;

## INGREDIENTS

- 1 orange, peeled, sliced
- 4 cups greens
- ½ of avocado, peeled, pitted, diced
- 2 tablespoons slivered red onion
- ½ cup cilantro

Extra:
- ¼ teaspoon salt
- ¼ cup olive oil
- 2 tablespoons lime juice
- 2 tablespoons orange juice

## DIRECTIONS

1. Prepare the dressing and for this, place cilantro in a food processor, pour in orange juice, lime juice, and oil, add salt and then pulse until blended.
2. Tip the dressing into a mason jar. Add remaining ingredients, toss until coated, and add to a salad bowl, or serve in jar.

# NOURISHING ELECTRIC SALAD

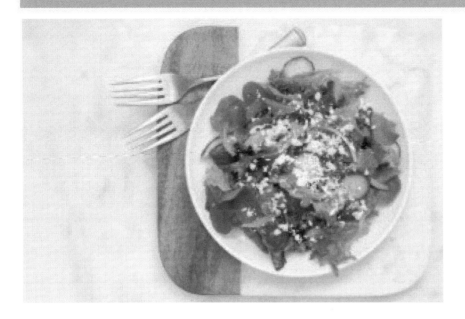

SERVING: 2

Preparation time: 5 minutes; Cooking time: 0 minutes;

NUTRITIONAL INFO: 129 Cal; 7 g Fats; 2 g Protein; 14 g Carb; 4 g Fiber;

## INGREDIENTS

- ½ of a medium cucumber, deseeded, chopped
- 6 leaves of lettuce, broke into pieces
- 4 mushrooms, chopped
- 6 cherry tomatoes, chopped
- 10 olives

Extra:
- ½ of lime, juiced
- 1 teaspoon olive oil
- ¼ teaspoon salt

## DIRECTIONS

1. Take a medium salad bowl, place all the ingredients in it and then toss until mixed.
2. Serve straight away.

# SUPERFOOD FONIO SALAD

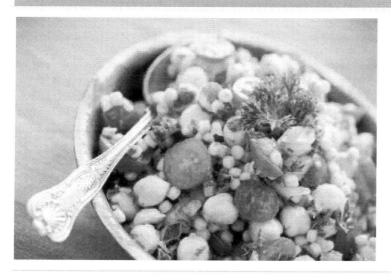

SERVING: 2; PREP TIME: 10 MINUTES; COOKING TIME: 5 MINUTES;

Nutritional Info: 145 Cal; 3 g Fats; 6 g Protein; 24.5 g Carb; 5.5 g Fiber;

## INGREDIENTS

- ½ cup cooked chickpeas
- ¼ cup chopped cucumber
- ½ cup chopped red pepper
- ½ cup cherry tomatoes, halved
- ½ cup fonio
- 1/3 teaspoon salt
- 1 tablespoon grapeseed oil
- 1/8 teaspoon cayenne pepper
- 1 key lime, juiced
- 1 cup spring water

## DIRECTIONS

1. Take a medium saucepan, place it over high heat, pour in water, and bring it to boil. Add fonio, switch heat to the low level, cook for 1 minute, and then remove the pan from heat.
2. Cover the pan with its lid, let fonio rest for 5 minutes, fluff by using a fork and then let it cool for 15 minutes.
3. Take a salad bowl, place lime juice and oil in it and then stir in salt and cayenne pepper until combined. Add remaining ingredients including fonio, toss until mixed, and then serve.

# HEALTHY CHICKPEA ROAST SALAD

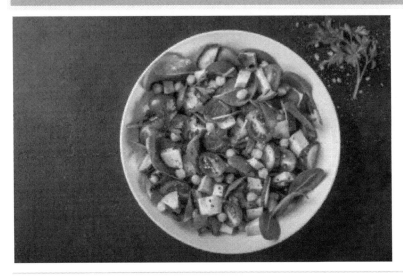

SERVING: 2; PREP TIME: 10 MINUTES; COOKING TIME: 20 MINUTES;

Nutritional Info: 208.3 Cal; 8 g Fats; 6.4 g Protein; 30 g Carb; 8 g Fiber;

## INGREDIENTS

- ½ of cucumber, deseeded, sliced
- 2 avocados, peeled, pitted, cubed
- 1 medium white onion, peeled, diced
- 2 cups cooked chickpeas
- ¼ cup chopped coriander
- 1 teaspoon onion powder
- ½ teaspoon cayenne pepper
- 1 teaspoon of sea salt
- 2 tablespoons hemp seeds, shelled
- 1 key lime, juiced
- 1 tablespoon olive oil

## DIRECTIONS

1. Switch on the oven, then set it to 425 degrees F and let it preheat.
2. Meanwhile, take a baking sheet, place chickpeas on it, season with salt, onion powder, and pepper, drizzle with oil and then toss until combined.
3. Bake the chickpeas for 20 minutes or until golden brown and crisp and then let them cool for 10 minutes.
4. Transfer chickpeas to a bowl, add remaining ingredients and stir until combined. Serve straight away.

# AMARANTH TABBOULEH SALAD

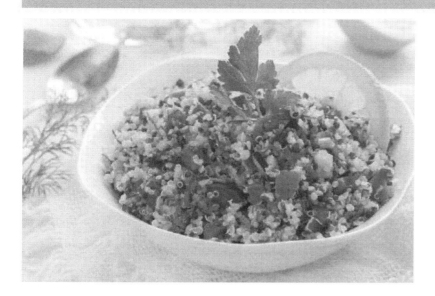

SERVING: 2

Preparation time: 5 minutes; Cooking time: 10 minutes;

Nutritional Info: 214 Cal; 4.5 g Fats; 6.5 g Protein; 37 g Carb; 9 g Fiber;

## INGREDIENTS

- 1 small white onion, peeled, chopped
- 1 cup cooked amaranth
- ½ of cucumber, deseeded, chopped
- 1 cup cooked chickpeas
- ½ of medium red bell pepper, chopped

Extra:
- 1/3 teaspoon sea salt
- 1/8 teaspoon cayenne pepper
- 2 tablespoons key lime juice

## DIRECTIONS

1. Take a small bowl, place lime juice in it, add salt and stir until combined.
2. Place remaining ingredients in a salad bowl, drizzle with lime juice mixture, toss until mixed, and then serve.

# DR. SEBI ZUCCHINI AND MUSHROOM BOWL

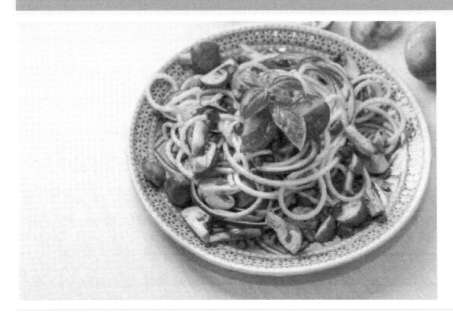

SERVING: 2

Preparation time: 5 minutes; Cooking time: 8 minutes;

Nutritional Info: 168 Cal; 2 g Fats; 0.9 g Protein; 36 g Carb; 6 g Fiber;

## INGREDIENTS

- 2 zucchini, spiralized
- ½ of medium red bell pepper, sliced
- ½ cup sliced mushrooms
- ½ of medium green bell pepper, sliced
- ½ of medium white onion, peeled, sliced

Extra:
- 1/3 teaspoon salt
- 1/8 teaspoon cayenne pepper
- 1 tablespoon grapeseed oil

## DIRECTIONS

1. Take a large skillet pan, place it over medium-high heat, add oil and when hot, add onion, mushrooms and bell peppers, and then cook for 3 to 5 minutes until tender-crisp.
2. Add zucchini noodles, toss until mixed, and then cook for 2 minutes until warm.
3. Serve straight away.

# SNACKS, APPETIZER AND MORE

## ALKALINE PEACH MUFFIN

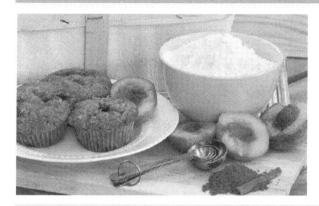

SERVING: 2; PREP TIME: 10 MINUTES; COOKING TIME: 15 MINUTES;

### INGREDIENTS

- 2/3 cup spelt flour; ½ of peach, chopped
- 1 teaspoon mashed burro banana
- 2/3 tablespoons chopped walnuts
- 6 ½ tablespoons walnut milk, homemade
- 1/16 teaspoon salt; 2 2/3 tablespoon date sugar
- 2/3 tablespoon spring water, warmed; 2/3 teaspoon key lime juice

### DIRECTIONS

1. Switch on the oven, then set it to 400 degrees F and let it preheat.
2. Meanwhile, peel the peach, cut it in half, remove the pit and then cut one half of peach in ½-inch pieces, reserving the other half of peach for later use.
3. Take a medium bowl, pour in the milk, and then whisk in mashed burro banana and lime juice until well combined.
4. Take a separate medium bowl, place flour in it, add salt and date sugar, stir until mixed, whisk in milk mixture until smooth, and then fold in peached until mixed.
5. Take four silicone muffin cups, grease them with oil, fill them evenly with the prepared batter and then sprinkle walnuts on top.
6. Bake the muffins for 10 to 15 minutes until the top is nicely golden brown and inserted toothpick into each muffin comes out clean.
7. When done, let muffins cool for 10 minutes and then serve.

# NUTTY BROWN ENERGY BALLS

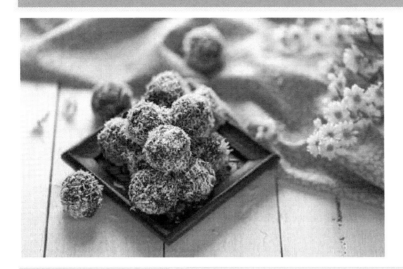

SERVING: 2

Preparation time: 10 minutes; Cooking time: 0 minutes;

Nutritional Info: 119 Cal; 8 g Fats; 2 g Protein; 10 g Carb; 1 g Fiber;

## INGREDIENTS

- ¼ cup blueberries
- ¼ cup dried dates
- 1 cup soft-jelly coconut, shredded
- ¼ cup walnuts
- ½ teaspoon date sugar

Extra:
- ½ tablespoon agave syrup
- 1/16 teaspoon salt

## DIRECTIONS

1. Place walnuts in a food processor and then pulse until the mixture resembles a fine powder.
2. Then add berries, coconut, date sugar and dates, pulse until just mixed and then slowly blend in agave syrup until the soft paste comes together.
3. Spoon the mixture into a medium bowl, chill it for a minimum of 30 minutes and then roll the mixture into balls, 1 tablespoon of mixture per ball.
4. Roll the balls into some more coconut and then serve.

# ZUCCHINI BREAD PANCAKES

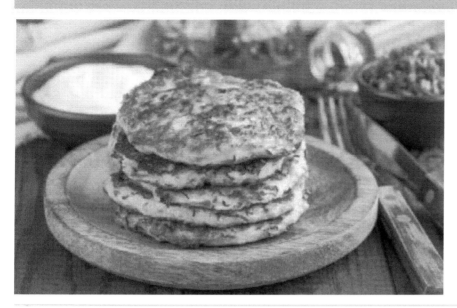

SERVING: 2

Preparation time: 10 minutes; Cooking time: 8 minutes;

Nutritional Info: 130 Cal; 4 g Fats; 3 g Protein; 21 g Carb; 3 g Fiber;

## INGREDIENTS

- 1 cup spelt flour
- ½ cup grated zucchini
- ¼ cup chopped walnuts
- 1 cup walnut milk, homemade

Extra:
- 1 tablespoon date sugar
- 1 tablespoon grapeseed oil

## DIRECTIONS

1. Take a medium bowl, place flour in it, add date sugar, and then stir until mixed.
2. Add mashed burro banana and milk in it, whisk until smooth batter comes together, and then fold in nuts and zucchini until just mixed.
3. Take a large skillet pan, place it over medium-high heat, add oil and when hot, pour the batter in it in portion and then shape each portion into a pancake.
4. Cook each pancake for 3 to 4 minutes per side and then serve.

## CHICKPEA NUGGETS

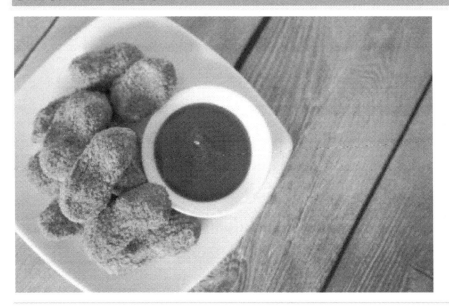

SERVING: 2

Preparation time: 10 minutes; Cooking time: 30 minutes;

Nutritional Info: 291.6 Cal; 3.9 g Fats; 19.9 g Protein; 26.8 g Carb; 3.4 g Fiber;

### INGREDIENTS

- 2 cups cooked chickpeas
- ½ teaspoon salt
- 1 teaspoon onion powder
- 1/3 cup and 1 tablespoon bread crumbs

### DIRECTIONS

1. Switch on the oven, then set it to 350 degrees F and let it preheat.
2. Meanwhile, place chickpeas in a food processor and then pulse until crumbled.
3. Tip the chickpeas in a bowl, add remaining ingredients in it except for 1/3 cup of breadcrumbs and then stir until a chunky mixture comes together.
4. Shape the mixture into evenly sized balls, shape each ball into the nugget, arrange on a baking sheet greased with oil and then bake for 15 minutes per side until golden brown.
5. Serve straight away.

# SPECIAL SPELT BANANA BREAD

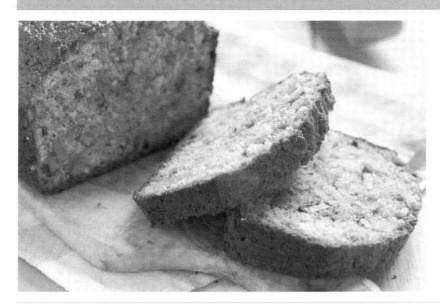

SERVING: 2

Preparation time: 10 minutes; Cooking time: 20 minutes;

Nutritional Info: 186 Cal; 11.3 g Fats; 1.3 g Protein; 22 g Carb; 2 g Fiber;

## INGREDIENTS

- 1/3 cup chopped walnuts
- 1 1/3 cup of burro banana
- 2/3 cup spelt flour
- 1/8 teaspoon salt
- ¼ cup agave syrup

Extra:
- 1 1/3 tablespoons olive oil

## DIRECTIONS

1. Switch on the oven, then set it to 350 degrees F and let it preheat.
2. Meanwhile, place the burro banana in a medium bowl, mash it by using a fork and then stir in oil and agave syrup until combined.
3. Take a separate medium bowl, place flour in it, add salt and nuts, stir until mixed, and then stir in the burro banana mixture until smooth.
4. Pour the batter into a parchment-lined loaf pan and then bake for 20 minutes until firm and the top turn golden brown.
5. When done, let the bread cool for 10 minutes, then cut it into slices and serve.

# INVIGORATING SEA MOSS PUDDING

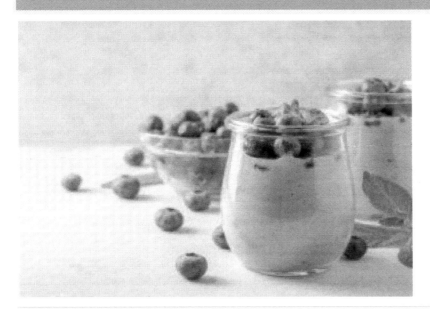

SERVING: 2

Preparation time: 5 minutes; Cooking time: 0 minutes;

Nutritional Info: 97.8 Cal; 0.5 g Fats; 0.7 g Protein; 23.4 g Carb; 2.8 g Fiber;

## INGREDIENTS

- 2 burro bananas, peeled
- 2 cups blueberries
- 6 tablespoons of sea moss gel
- ½ cup spring Water

## DIRECTIONS

1. Plug in a high-speed food processor or blender and add all the ingredients in its jar except for water.
2. Cover the blender jar with its lid, pulse until smooth, and then slowly blend in water until thickened to the desire level.
3. Serve straight away.

# DELICIOUS AVOCADO TOMATO TOAST

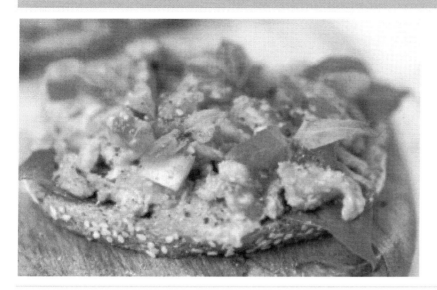

SERVING: 2

Preparation time: 5 minutes; Cooking time: 0 minutes;

Nutritional Info: 189 Cal; 11 g Fats; 3 g Protein; 20 g Carb; 5.4 g Fiber;

## INGREDIENTS

- 2 slices of spelt bread, toasted
- 1 avocado, peeled, pitted, mashed
- ½ cup cherry tomato halves
- ½ teaspoon salt
- 2 teaspoons key lime juice

## DIRECTIONS

1. Place avocado in a bowl, add lime juice, and then mash until smooth.
2. Spread mashed avocado evenly on top of each toast and then scatter cherry tomatoes.
3. Sprinkle salt over tomatoes and then serve.

# TASTY RYE CRACKERS

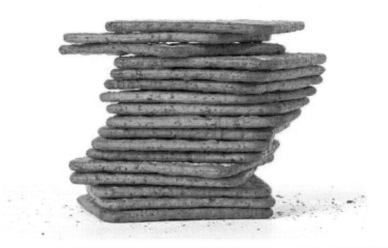

## SERVING: 2

Preparation time: 10 minutes; Cooking time: 10 minutes;

Nutritional Info: 81.2 Cal; 1.2 g Fats; 0.8 g Protein; 16.4 g Carb; 1.7 g Fiber;

## INGREDIENTS

- 1 cup rye flour
- 1 teaspoon onion powder
- ½ teaspoon salt
- ½ teaspoon dried thyme
- ½ teaspoon dried basil
- 2 tablespoons grapeseed oil
- 4 tablespoons spring water

## DIRECTIONS

1. Switch on the oven, then set it to 400 degrees F and let it preheat.
2. Meanwhile, place flour in a food processor, add all the seasonings and oil, and then pulse until combined.
3. Add water, pulse until the dough comes together, and then roll it into a ½-inch thick dough.
4. Use a cookie cutter of the desired shape to cut out cookie, arrange them on a large baking sheet and then bake for 10 minutes until nicely browned. Serve straight away.

# SOUPS, STEWS AND SAUCES

## ZOODLE VEGETABLE SOUP

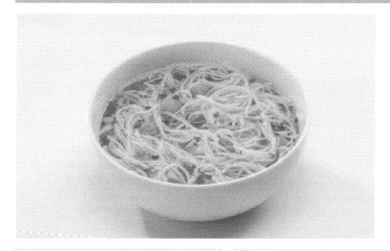

SERVING: 2

Preparation time: 5 minutes; Cooking time: 12 minutes;

Nutritional Info: 265 Cal; 2 g Fats; 4 g Protein; 57 g Carb; 13.6 g Fiber;

INGREDIENTS

- ½ of onion, peeled, cubed
- ½ of green bell pepper, chopped
- ½ of zucchini, grated
- 4 ounces sliced mushrooms, chopped
- ½ cup cherry tomatoes
- ¼ cup basil leaves
- 1 pack of spelt noodles, cooked
- ¼ teaspoon salt
- 1/8 teaspoon cayenne pepper
- ½ of key lime, juiced
- 1 tablespoon grapeseed oil
- 2 cups spring water

DIRECTIONS

1. Take a medium saucepan, place it over medium heat, add oil and when hot, add onion and then cook for 3 minutes or more until tender.
2. Add cherry tomatoes, bell pepper, and mushrooms, stir until mixed, and then continue cooking for 3 minutes until soft.

3. Add grated zucchini, season with salt, cayenne pepper, pour in the water, and then bring the mixture to a boil.
4. Then switch heat to the low level, add cooked noodles and then simmer the soup for 5 minutes.
5. When done, ladle soup into two bowls, top with basil leaves, drizzle with lime juice and then serve.

## CUCUMBER AND BASIL GAZPACHO

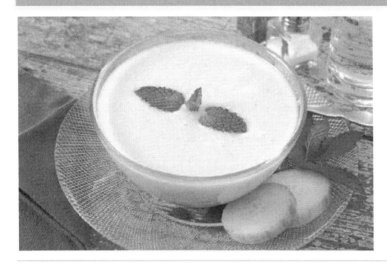

SERVING: 2

Preparation time: 5 minutes; Cooking time: 0 minutes;

Nutritional Info: 190 Cal; 15 g Fats; 4 g Protein; 15 g Carb; 6 g Fiber;

### INGREDIENTS

- 1 avocado, peeled, pitted, cold
- 1 cucumber, deseeded, unpeeled, cold
- ½ cup basil leaves, cold
- ½ of key lime, juiced
- 2 cups spring water, chilled

Extra:
- 1 ½ teaspoon sea salt

### DIRECTIONS

1. Place all the ingredients into the jar of a high-speed food processor or blender and then pulse until smooth.
2. Tip the soup into a medium bowl and then chill for a minimum of 1 hour.

3. Divide the soup evenly between two bowls, top with some more basil and then serve.

## SPICY SOURSOP AND ZUCCHINI SOUP

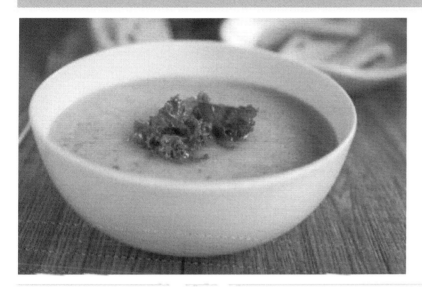

SERVING: 2

Preparation time: 5 minutes; Cooking time: 45 minutes;

Nutritional Info: 224 Cal; 5 g Fats; 5.8 g Protein; 38.1 g Carb; 3.4 g Fiber;

### INGREDIENTS

- 1 cup chopped kale
- 2 Soursop leaves, rinsed, rip in half
- ½ cup summer squash cubes
- 1 cup chayote squash cubes
- ½ cup zucchini cubes

Extra:
- ½ cup wild rice
- ½ cup diced white onions
- 1 cup diced green bell peppers
- 2 teaspoons sea salt
- ½ tablespoon basil
- ¼ teaspoon cayenne pepper
- ½ tablespoon oregano
- 6 cups spring water

### DIRECTIONS

1. Take a medium pot, place it over medium-high heat, add soursop leaves, pour in 1 ½ cup water, and then boil for 15 minutes, covering the pan with lid.
2. When done, remove eaves from the broth, switch heat to medium level, add remaining ingredients into the pot, stir until mixed, and then cook for 30 minutes or more until done.
3. Serve straight away.

## DELICIOUS CHICKPEA & MUSHROOM BOWL

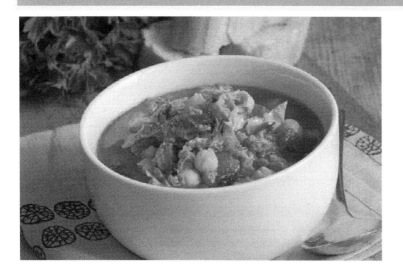

SERVING: 2

Preparation time: 5 minutes; Cooking time: 10 minutes;

Nutritional Info: 242 Cal; 9 g Fats; 10 g Protein; 34 g Carb; 9 g Fiber;

INGREDIENTS

- 1 ½ cup cooked chickpeas
- 2 zucchinis, spiralized
- 4 small oyster mushrooms, destemmed, diced
- ¼ of white onion, peeled, chopped
- ¼ of red bell pepper, cored, chopped

Extra:
- 1/3 teaspoon sea salt; 1 teaspoon dried basil
- ¼ teaspoon cayenne pepper; 1 teaspoon dried oregano
- 1 tablespoon grapeseed oil
- 2 ½ cups vegetable broth, homemade

## DIRECTIONS

1. Take a medium pot, place it over medium-high heat, add oil and when hot, add red pepper, onion, and mushrooms, season with salt and cayenne pepper, and then cook for 5 minutes until tender.
2. Switch heat to medium-low level, add remaining ingredients except for zucchini noodles, stir until mixed, and then simmer the soup for 15 to 20 minutes.
3. Then add zucchini noodles into the pan, stir until mixed, and then cook for 1 minute or more until thoroughly warmed. Serve straight away.

# ZOODLE CHICKPEA SOUP

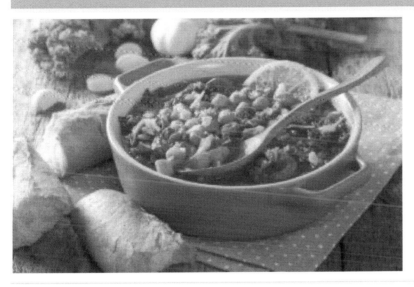

SERVING: 2

Preparation time: 5 minutes; Cooking time: 25 minutes;

Nutritional Info: 184.5 Cal; 0.3 g Fats; 6.8 g Protein; 31 g Carb; 6 g Fiber;

## INGREDIENTS

- ½ cup cooked, chickpeas
- ½ of a medium white onion, peeled, diced
- ½ of a large zucchini, chopped
- 1 cup kale leaves
- 1 cup squash cubes

Extra:
- ¾ teaspoon salt
- ¾ tablespoon chopped thyme, fresh

- ¾ tablespoon tarragon, fresh
- 2 cups vegetable broth, homemade
- 1 ½ cup spring water

## DIRECTIONS

1. Take a saucepan, place it over medium-high heat, pour in the ¼ cup broth, add zucchini, onion, and thyme and then cook for 4 minutes.
2. Pour in remaining broth and water, bring it to a boil, switch heat to the low level, and then simmer for 10 to 15 minutes until tender.
3. Add remaining ingredients, stir until mixed, and then continue cooking for 10 minutes or more until cooked.
4. Serve straight away.

# OTHER BOOKS IN SAME SERIES

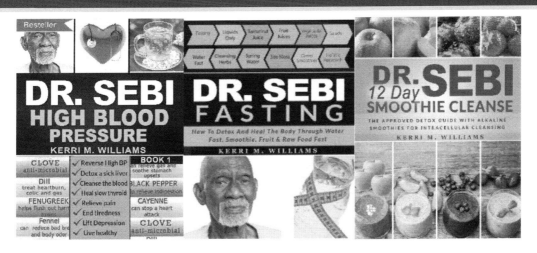

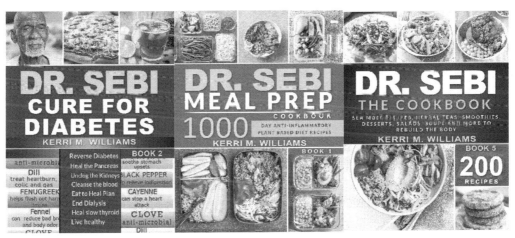

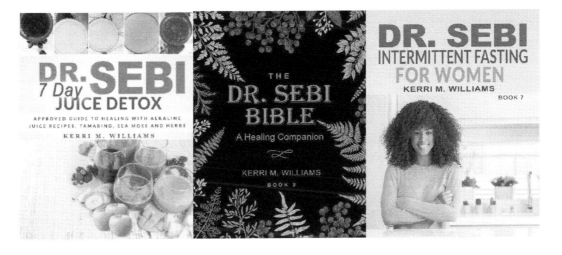

Made in the USA
Columbia, SC
20 November 2021

49408573R00122